Praise for

BE *GOOD* TO YOUR *BODY*

"In her newest and most profound work to date, *Be Good to Your Body*, Jordan has taken historical biblical truths and translated them into daily, practical, healthy rhythms that, when implemented, will allow each of us to build and sustain the lives—and bodies—we really want to have. To the glory of God."

—ANNIE F. DOWNS, *New York Times* bestselling author of
That Sounds Fun

"Another outstanding effort by Jordon Lee Dooley. Better than anyone else I've read, she asks and answers the difficult question 'What is health and how do I get it?' This book is guaranteed to improve your approach to managing both your emotional and physical wellness."

—CHRISTOPHER STROUD, MD

"Today, as women, it can be confusing to know how to live healthy, embodied lives. It's easy to swing from one extreme to another—or to stay apathetic because we're not sure what's true or best. Jordan invites us in with her own vulnerable story and sets our gaze back on Jesus. She cuts through all the confusion by offering wisdom and knowledge of how to actually live a healthy life that is attainable and full of freedom and joy."

—ALYSSA JOY BETHKE, author of *When Do It All Is Undoing You*
and *Satisfied*

"*Be Good to Your Body* is groundbreaking, shame silencing, and grace filled. It's anointed—instructing and encouraging us on every page to not just be good stewards of our God-given bodies but also to take joy in them. If you're tired of worldly, superficial advice on your body and wellness journey, Jordan has the biblical wisdom and practical truth you're looking for."

—TARA SUN, author of *Overbooked and Overwhelmed* and host of the *Truth Talks with Tara* podcast

"Our bodies are brilliantly designed by a wonderful creator. The human race has complicated this issue over time, but Jordan's approach in *Be Good to Your Body* is simple yet profound: 'What does Scripture say about it?' This question should guide *any* topic a believer explores but especially when considering what true health is (and is not). This message is so important in our social media generation: Tune out the noise and go back to the way God designed us to eat, think, and live. As a mom of six, I can confidently say this book will benefit all female believers who wish to honor the Lord with the body He has given them. The wisdom Jordan has gained through her experiences—and so graciously shared in these pages— will be a source of insight and inspiration for all who read this book."

—ELIZABETH PARSONS, creator, founder of Purely Parsons

"*Be Good to Your Body* feels like a late-night chat with a best friend. It's a compelling conversation about how to counterculturally choose to put Christ on the throne of health rather than self. Jordan provides both a thoughtful reflection on her own journey and practical steps toward wisely stewarding our God-given bodies. You'll set this book down feeling encouraged to be truly nourished—body and soul. And maybe . . . you just need a nap and a snack."

—KRISTEN VAN GILSE, The OrganiMama

"With empathy, honesty, and grace, Jordan Lee Dooley not only guides us on how to steward our bodies well, but she also sheds light on *why* doing so matters a great deal. While directing our attention to the God who made our bodies, she compels us to live by a definition of 'health' that contrasts the variety of ways culture has defined it. *Be Good to Your Body* is timely, beneficial, and relatable. I am grateful for these words."

—EMMA MAE MCDANIEL, author of *The Girl in the Middle*

BE *GOOD*
TO YOUR
BODY

BE *GOOD* TO YOUR *BODY*

GETTING BACK TO GOD'S DESIGN IN A WORLD
OF WELLNESS TRENDS, QUICK FIXES, AND
CONFLICTING HEALTH ADVICE

Jordan Lee Dooley

FOREWORD BY
Annika Robinson,
Functional Nutritional Therapy Practitioner

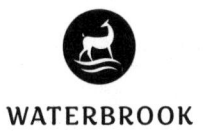

WATERBROOK

WaterBrook
An imprint of the Penguin Random House Christian Publishing Group,
a division of Penguin Random House LLC
1745 Broadway, New York, NY 10019
waterbrookmultnomah.com
penguinrandomhouse.com

LIBRARY OF CONGRESS CATALOGING-IN-PUBLICATION DATA
Names: Dooley, Jordan Lee author
Title: Be good to your body: getting back to god's design in a world of wellness trends, quick fixes, and
conflicting health advice / Jordan Lee Dooley.
Description: First edition. | New York, NY: WaterBrook, [2025] | Includes bibliographical references.
Identifiers: LCCN 2025008181 | ISBN 9780593193471 hardcover | ISBN 9780593193488 ebook
Subjects: LCSH: Christian women—Religious life | Health—Religious aspects—Christianity
Classification: LCC BV4527 .D659 2025 | DDC 364—dc23/eng/20250703
LC record available at https://lccn.loc.gov/2025008181

Printed in the United States of America on acid-free paper

2nd Printing

First Edition

The authorized representative in the EU for product safety and compliance is
Penguin Random House Ireland, Morrison Chambers, 32 Nassau Street,
Dublin D02 YH68, Ireland. https://eu-contact.penguin.ie

BOOK TEAM: Editor: Susan Tjaden • Production editor: Helen Macdonald • Managing editor:
Julia Wallace • Production manager: Meghan O'Leary • Copy editor: Cara Iverson • Proofreaders:
Bailey Utecht, Carrie Krause, Marissa Earl

Book design by Alexis Flynn

Interior illustrations by Sophie Konop

For details on special quantity discounts for bulk purchases,
contact specialmarketscms@penguinrandomhouse.com.

For my children, who have inspired me
to be good to my body even before you were born.

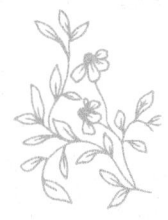

FOREWORD

Like many modern-day friendships, Jordan and I met through Instagram. We connected right away over the similarities of our health journeys. Reading her words in this book about her past health struggles made me feel as though I were reliving my own story. Maybe you have experienced—or are currently going through—something similar.

"Can you believe we used to suffer from these problems and then take such harmful and extreme actions to try to heal?" I texted Jordan as I was reading through the chapters. It made me sad to reminisce on how lost, scared, and broken we both felt before we discovered the truth about how God designed us to eat and live. Jordan's past, like mine, was riddled with physical pain and emotional heartache due to endometriosis diagnoses, adult acne, body dysmorphia, and more.

Jordan and I didn't just connect because of our pasts and the difficulties we had faced with our health; more important, we deeply identified with each other on our beliefs as to how the body heals and thrives.

What Jordan has discovered through her own journey, and what she's shared with us in *Be Good to Your Body,* is what I've been shouting from the rooftops for years. You don't need to be a registered dietitian or holistic nutritionist or have some sort of certification or letters behind your name to figure this out. What you need is the desire to turn back to the wisdom the Lord has shared with us in the Bible, which Jordan communicates so perfectly in this book. This ancient wisdom, given to us by God Himself, supersedes any fifty-ingredient anti-aging serum or bio hack or restrictive diet that our social media feed tells us we absolutely need.

Jordan did the deep work while she was on her journey, which she shared so well in *Be Good to Your Body.* She opened her Bible and asked a very important question: *How am I really supposed to care for myself as a woman living in modern society and also following Jesus?* And the conclusions she came to are the exact ones that I have.

As a functional nutritional therapy practitioner, I've helped thousands of women of all ages heal from a wide array of debilitating issues. You'd think I'd have made some breakthrough discovery on what all women are lacking—some pearl of wisdom or eureka moment of figuring out what particular supplement, nutrient, or vitamin every woman is missing. But in that time, I've made only one major discovery. It's that women—of all ages and walks of life—are *confused* when it comes to health, beauty, and femininity and simply need to be redirected to the truth. That's it.

By no fault of our own, we've come so incredibly far from understanding what true health, true beauty, and true femininity look like. Society and the enormous industries that spend billions of dollars marketing to us are all selling us the same idea: that women's bodies are inherently broken and need some magic solution or quick fix.

When you think about it, that is exactly what the Enemy wants. After all, he is the Father of Lies and would love nothing more than to make us feel isolated. He wants you to feel like you are the only woman lost, broken, and confused—alone on a path of "dis-ease" and frustration with your body.

We're sick and exhausted as women not because we're not doing enough, not because we're not working out enough, and certainly not because we haven't eliminated enough foods or carbs from our diets. We're sick because we are being deceived, and it's time to end this pattern of deception once and for all.

Be Good to Your Body could not have addressed and cleared up this confusion and deception more perfectly. As a reader of this book, you will feel seen, heard, and known. And furthermore, you'll start to understand your body and your femininity for perhaps the very first time.

That is why I believe *Be Good to Your Body* isn't just another good book for women of all ages. In fact, it is *critical* for all of us female believers to read and benefit from the wisdom inside its pages. As Jordan illustrates, it is actually quite simple to be good to our bodies. We don't need another product or diet; rather, we need to get back to the way God designed us to eat and live.

Jordan has made a very important discovery in this book, which is that God created us to thrive and gave us what we need to do so. He truly wants us to be good to and respect our bodies, which He fearfully and wonderfully made. That is the only way health is truly possible.

Jordan illustrates for us how the Bible repeatedly points us to the importance of caring for our bodies. Why is that so important, and why is that theme prevalent throughout Scripture? As you'll read, it's so we can fulfill our individual callings as women. Each of us has unique spiritual gifts (see Romans 12:6–8). We are called to serve the Lord by being His hands and feet and to spread the gospel through our unique talents. How can we do that when we are chronically ill and fatigued and just don't feel well?

Let's use Jordan's story—and this book itself—as an example of how that can look. She felt as though her body was failing her, and she couldn't think about much else beyond getting better by *fixing it*. Her femininity was wounded by the Enemy's lies she faced when she was suffering from acne, fertility issues, and pregnancy loss (the biggest fear of any woman who longs to be a mother). But God had bigger plans for Jordan—and for me *and for you*.

The very fact that *Be Good to Your Body* exists is a testament to the faithfulness of our Father and the healing that can happen when we live according to His will. Because of Jordan's healing and all that she learned in the process, and because she feels good enough to share her gifts with the world, we now have a book that can help the many thousands of women who will glean the wisdom from its pages.

God, we know that none of us will experience perfect health or a pain-free life outside of heaven. Please bless the readers of this book and help them take this wisdom to heart, implement the changes, and begin reclaiming their health so they can share their unique and beautiful gifts with the world. With the help from teachings in this book, please help us build lives that help us return to the way You designed us to eat and live, so we can expand Your kingdom. Amen.

In health and God's blessings,
Annika Robinson, FNTP, EMT, birth doula

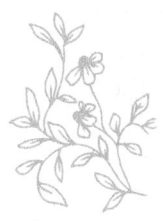

CONTENTS

BE *GOOD* TO YOUR *BODY*

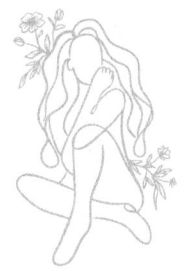

Chapter One

HOW DID WE GET HERE?

I wish you and I were sitting together, sipping adrenal mocktails by a cozy fire at a little bungalow in the mountains somewhere far away, because if you picked up this book, I think we'd have a lot to talk about. We'd probably find a thing or two (or twelve) in common.

But since we can't do that, we'll just have to discuss things through these pages. And as much as I'd love to hear about your own journey with health and wellness, for now I'll just share some of my story here, because I bet some of it will resonate with you. Before I dig in, let me cover why we're even here together.

It's time to have a conversation about how we're treating our bodies. The women of the modern world we live in have become experts in restricting, treating, and manipulating our bodies in pursuit of a cultural standard of health or beauty. Sometimes both. I don't know how old you are, but I'm in my thirties—which means I'm part of the generation who grew up wearing Bath & Body

Works body spray while consuming mostly low-fat and low-calorie everything. We saw the endless ads for Jenny Craig, Slim-Fast, and WeightWatchers, geared toward women everywhere. Even some of our eighty-something-year-old grandmas commented on how they'd put on weight. Apparently, body fixation doesn't even end at eighty!

Then . . . *whiplash!* . . . we were hit with the body-positivity movement, where we were told that no matter what size or shape our bodies are, we should just love them.

We live in a time when convenience food (hot dogs, anyone?) and food-like products (hello, margarine and Kraft Mac & Cheese) are seemingly more available and affordable than real, nutrient-dense food. Many of us wouldn't know how to source food or what to do if it weren't for the grocery store and DoorDash.

And the challenge goes beyond just the food we eat. For example, we were conditioned to believe that birth control was the solution to countless symptoms known to trouble the female body *and* the key to achieving our wildest dreams, all without being well educated on potential downsides or side effects.

We've lived a good part of our adult lives being bombarded by conflicting health advice about diet culture (many of us restricting or meticulously counting calories in our teen and young adult years), body positivity (love your body at any size), intuitive eating (stop thinking about different foods as "good" or "bad"), biohacking (wearable fitness gadgets, apps, cold plunging, and more), and popular healing diets advertised all over Instagram (follow Whole30 or Paleo). Many of those ideas hold some good, but in our information age, it can be not only overwhelming but also difficult to discern where to start or what to focus on.

And that's why we're here: to unlearn all the ways we've complicated healthy living and reclaim what it really means to be good to our bodies, *biblically* and *holistically*, because many of us were once sold this big lie:

$$\text{HEALTH} = \begin{array}{l}\text{cutting calories + waking up at 5:00 A.M. to work out} \\ \text{+ masking symptoms + taking a thousand vitamins +} \\ \text{being extremely lean}\end{array}$$

And then we began to realize that perhaps that was not at all good for our hormones, fertility, or bodies. So the world sold us the idea that *self-love* and *body positivity* were the solution to all that we'd been conditioned to believe.

But is that actually a solution? Or is it just daring us to swing to the opposite extreme, where "loving yourself" can lead to carelessness, lack of moderation, and even neglect of essential aspects to a healthy body, such as intentional exercise, fresh air, adequate rest, hydration, and quality nutrition?

What if the real solution to these extremes of diet culture and body positivity has been there all along, nestled in the pages of the Bible—the Word of the One who created our bodies to begin with and the only book that reveals how we were designed and what our bodies have truly needed to thrive since the beginning of time? What if we trusted that God is smarter than we are? Smarter than our cool slogans and graphics and movements and diets and fancy studies? What if He's given us the guidelines for what it means to be healthy, care for our natural beauty, and be good to our bodies?

What if we've been so wrapped up with the latest health hacks that we've missed what it means to actually be healthy? We've been flooded with new information and studies and gurus and diets and wellness gadgets and trends for so long. No wonder we're confused and tired. Trying to keep up with the world's ever-changing idea of healthy living is exhausting.

But maybe it's not as complicated as we've made it. In fact, maybe it's really simple.

YOUR BODY IS A GOD-GIVEN GIFT, NOT A PROJECT TO FIX

I don't know about you, but there have been several times in my life when I viewed fitness or wellness as a way to "fix" my body. Can you relate?

At one point, my pursuit of health and wellness was driven by a desire to *look* a certain way. In college, I embarked on a fitness journey, striving to achieve six-pack abs and a slimmer waist. I was obsessed with the scale and got into a vicious cycle of overexercising and undereating, all in the pursuit of what I thought would make me more attractive. And admittedly, I was seeking *control* during a time when much felt new and unfamiliar. Counting calories, completing workouts, and logging miles felt like something I could control.

Now in my thirties, I wish I could go back to myself at nineteen or twenty and tell her to cool it on overexercising, obsessive calorie counting, and relying on copious amounts of caffeine for energy. I wish I could tell her to instead support her body with gentle movement, adequate rest, and real nourishment. I would tell her to replenish her body with the good things God created rather than trying to restrict the "bad things" the fitness world deems unhealthy (like carbs and calories), because all those habits were going to destroy her hormonal health and thyroid before she knew it.

Sigh. My mom tried to tell me, but I didn't want to listen.

Anyway, a handful of years later, I had toned it down a bit on the excessive exercise and calorie counting but *still* thought I was the picture of health because I drank green juice, worked out almost daily, and managed to stay fairly lean. That's what the world around me said was healthy, anyway. But if I was so healthy, why did I have such heavy periods and horrible PMS? Why was my skin being taken over by cystic acne when I was well over a decade removed from puberty? And why was my "young and healthy" body unable to carry a baby to term, resulting in recurring miscarriages?

I wanted answers. I needed solutions. I was young and *healthy . . .* right? Why was this happening to me?

I started digging, determined to find root causes. I looked for anything I could find that might help improve my situation and heal the symptoms I was experiencing. I found lots of supplements and naturopaths and Whole30 and chiropractic care and Paleo and a million and one other things. I joined a dozen healthy-living Facebook groups and researched like a madwoman everything I could find on hormones and fertility and gut health.

See, this time around, I wasn't so concerned with *form* as I was with *function.* I didn't mind so much if I wasn't my thinnest or fittest; I just wanted my body to work how it was supposed to. I wanted my skin to be like that of an adult and not a teenage girl. I wanted to wake up with natural energy. And more than anything, I wanted my body to do what it was designed to do: bring forth life.

I was on a mission to fix my body.

Inherently, seeking answers and root causes rather than just slapping a Band-Aid on symptoms is a good thing. But somewhere along the way, I stopped viewing my body as a God-given gift and instead began to see it as a project to fix.

I started with good intentions—I wanted to take better care of my health, steward my body, and support my fertility naturally—but even the best of intentions can begin to spiral into obsession.

And for me, that looked like restrictive "healing" diets, a thousand supplements, and trying to remove every last toxin from my life in an effort to fix whatever was wrong with me.

I made some progress and saw improvement in some ways, but as I researched more and more, I also began to feel confused by all the health advice and insight I was hearing. So much of the information I consumed was conflicting, from different schools of thought on things like dairy to the absence of a real definition of what makes a product "clean."

Eventually, I began to get burned-out trying to get healthy all on my own and taking advice from the world. I stepped back for a bit and realized I had been listening to so many voices but had failed to consider the voice of the One who created my body in the first place. I had read a slew of studies and books on health and naturally healing the body, but I never really thought to consider how the Bible—the book that details how our bodies were designed and what was initially made for them to thrive from the beginning of time—might have some of the answers I was looking for.

I had unintentionally shut God out of my health journey—or at least I didn't invite Him in. I didn't partner with Him as I sought to understand and support my body.

Don't get me wrong. I had a spiritual life. I went to church and read the Bible, listened to worship music, and was plugged into a great community. But somewhere in my brain, I had separated the spiritual from the physical. I kind of forgot that although scientists, doctors, and studies have tons of helpful information on health and healing, the One who came up with the idea of humanity in the first place *miiiiight* know a thing or two about supporting a healthy body.

I hope you're picking up on my sarcasm here, because the God of all creation definitely knows more than any human being, and perhaps it'd do us some good to partner with Him in our pursuit of health and healing.

As I realized those things, I asked myself a few questions:

- *Have I turned a good thing (my body) into a god thing?*
- *Has wellness become an idol? Has a good intention spiraled into an obsession?*
- *What does the Bible say? And what did God create for my body to thrive?*
- *How can I focus on living in alignment with God's design rather than getting tangled up in all the world's trends and health advice?*

Those questions helped me examine my heart and course correct a bit. And by "course correct," I don't mean swinging to the opposite extreme and abandoning my health journey altogether. Rather, I began making sure my pursuit of healing and well-being was from a place of obedience and freedom and not of obsession and fear.

I loosened my tight grip. I focused on areas I could prioritize. I ignored most of the random advice I was seeing online and went back to the basic principles of health that God laid out in Genesis when He created us.

And guess what happened?

In time, my skin began to clear, my energy improved, and I even had a baby. When I stopped attempting to do it all on my own, when I stopped trying so hard to fix my body and instead focused on *being good to my body*—on considering my biological needs, giving my body the good things God designed for it to thrive, and seeking out help in the areas in which I needed additional support—it actually began to be good to me.

Huh. Imagine that. We've complicated healthy living so much in our society of quick fixes, convenience, fads, and endless information (and opinions) that it's no wonder we're confused and exhausted. But it's actually pretty simple.

So what I want to explore together is this: How can we be good to our bodies—biblically *and* practically—in a world of trends, confusing advice online, and extremes (like diet culture and self-love)? After all, it's far too easy to begin to live at one end of the spectrum or the other when it comes to how we care for our bodies. We often see examples of *idolatry* (being obsessed with health and healthy living) or *idleness* (loving our bodies as they are, with little regard for what is actually good for them).

It's like either we're all in (meticulously counting calories, overexercising, and obsessing over avoiding every possible toxin) *or* we're just being somewhat passive about it all, running the risk of not making any effort to be better stewards under the guise of *self-love* or *body positivity* or whatever other label we slap on it.

But we have to talk about this because the biblical view of the body directly affects how we care for it. Unfortunately, even Christians tend to separate the physical and the spiritual, as if they can be separated. But is that what the Bible teaches?

Romans 12:1 says that our *bodies* were meant to be living sacrifices, holy and acceptable to God, for this is our *spiritual* act of worship.

The two cannot be separated.

I love how Nancy Pearcey puts it in her book *Love Thy Body:* "Christianity holds that body and soul together form an integrated unity—that the human being is an embodied soul."[1] She goes on to say, "If the body has no intrinsic purpose, built in by God, then all that matters are human purposes.... It is raw material to be manipulated and controlled to serve the human agenda, like any other natural resource."[2]

First, that means that neglecting the body is considered neglect of the entire being. It also means that obsessing over perfecting the body (in terms of either form, function, or both) that lives in a broken world can quickly turn into trying to manipulate or control the body for our own purposes.

Another wise woman, Elisabeth Elliot, says, "[It is a failure not] to recognize this living body as having anything to do with worship or holy sacrifice. This body is, quite simply, the starting place. Failure here is failure everywhere else."[3]

It all starts with the body. If we want to be well holistically (meaning spiritually, emotionally, and mentally), we start with the body—with being good to the body and giving it the good things God made—without making the body a god.

THE REMEDY TO IDOLATRY AND APATHY

Wait, what do I mean by "making the body a god"?

When wellness or the body becomes an idol (the object of our worship), it's nearly impossible to be holistically well, because both obsession and striving for perfection lead to stress. And stress takes a toll not only on the physical body but also on emotional, mental, and spiritual well-being. As I mentioned, the world has suggested that practicing self-love and body positivity is the secret to being good to our bodies. But is it? Are we healthier *holistically*?

The answer is no, we are not. For proof, let's look at some data.

First, a 2023 Gallup survey revealed that 17.8 percent of adults in the United States have a diagnosis of depression, which is an all-time high.[4] And according to the Centers for Disease Control and Prevention (CDC), the prevalence of chronic diseases has been increasing steadily over the past two decades. An estimated 129 million people in the United States have at least one major chronic disease, such as heart disease, cancer, diabetes, obesity, and hypertension.[5]

What's more, according to *The Washington Post,* American life expectancy is dropping due to chronic health conditions, despite our country having some of the most advanced medical care in the world.[6]

We have more self-love than ever and simultaneously have more mental health and chronic health issues than ever. I'm not claiming that self-love is to blame, but my question is, If it were really helping, wouldn't we see an improvement in the way our collective mental or physical health is trending?

Plus, our natural human default position is to focus on the self—to view ourselves as the main character in our own stories. We already think about ourselves constantly. Virtually everything we do revolves around making ourselves look better and being more comfortable.

I would argue that our natural focus is *already* on ourselves—meeting our own needs, desires, and passions—and it is for that very reason why things like motherhood and marriage can be so beautifully challenging. Those roles force us to repeatedly set aside our self-centered inclinations for the sake of others. Yet as we learn to lay down our lives as the Bible teaches us, many find serving others—whether spouses, children, or someone else—to be the most fulfilling thing they've ever done.

In the Bible, 2 Timothy 3:1–2 warns that one of the characteristics of the "last days" will be people who are "lovers of self." And Scripture never instructs us to practice self-love. Self-love as the world defines it will always come up short because the answers and peace we seek cannot be found in the self. The purpose and peace that we desire can be found only outside ourselves: in the One who formed us and breathed life into us.

So, what's the solution we're really looking for? Is it simpler than we've made it out to be? Quite possibly.

Biblically (and practically) speaking, stewardship is the key to being truly good to our bodies. *Stewardship* is a word I have heard most of my life but for a long time either overlooked or just poorly understood. Maybe you can relate? So in the pages that follow, let's explore what it *does* mean.

WHAT IS STEWARDSHIP?

Last summer, I was at a backyard graduation party, catching up with a friend. She was finally pregnant after years of infertility and a miscarriage. I could relate since my own journey to motherhood had been challenging, and I knew how hard it can be to embrace and celebrate a pregnancy after loss and infertility. It just feels like you're constantly waiting for the other shoe to drop.

We chatted about this a bit, and then she said, "It's really the ultimate test of stewardship."

Wait, what? I thought. *Stewardship?* I expected her to say *surrender, trust,* or *faith.* But *stewardship*? What did she mean by that?

I cocked my head, as if to ask her to explain.

"I mean, yeah," she continued as she turned her open palms up to the sky. "It's like, everything I have is Yours, Lord. Even my body. And my people."

Yes! That *is what stewardship is.*

It was truly the simplest yet most accurate description of stewardship I'd ever heard. Stewardship is about not just what you *do* but ultimately what you *believe,* because what you believe—about God, your body, and any other blessing—directly influences how you do anything.

Think about it this way: If a friend gave me her car to use, I would take the very best care of it. I wouldn't obsess over the car's condition or fixate on any flaw, such as a ding or scratch it may have had when she loaned it to me. But I would care for it well. Wouldn't you? Wouldn't you drive with both hands on the wheel, keep your eyes on the road, pay close attention to where you parked, make sure to give it the right kind of fuel, and keep it clean instead of letting junk pile up in the passenger seat?

> What you believe—about God, your body, and any other blessing—directly influences how you do anything.

It may help to think of our bodies like that car. In today's world, it can be so easy to forget that biblically even our bodies (and our babies) are not our own to do with whatever we please.

I know that may step on some toes, but it's kind of freeing when you think about it.

Our bodies are kind of like that borrowed car: beautiful gifts from God, given to us as vehicles to carry out our callings during our short time on earth.

For that reason alone, we should take utmost care of our bodies. Not obsess over them. Not critique them or pick them apart or treat them as projects to fix. But we should care for them because they are sacred gifts. Stewardship is a palms-up, surrendered-heart posture that says, "Everything I have is Yours," and treating it accordingly.

When we view everything we have as our creator's, we care for it differently.

Let's go back to the car example for a minute. I'm much more likely to let my own car get messy, drive it with a nearly empty tank, or put off that oil change it needs. Not because I don't care or am trying to be irresponsible, but because life is busy and when something is my own, there's little to no accountability. But when it's my friend's car? I treat that car with the utmost respect, care, and concern. Not because I love the car, but because *I love my friend* and want to honor and respect the gift she's giving me.

On the other hand, when I care for my friend's car, is it because I *hate* the car? Because I think it's ugly and needs to be fixed? No, I care for it because *I love my friend* and appreciate what she has given me.

The point is that the gift is good, but it is not what is ultimately important to me. My relationship with the one who gave it to me is. And part of how I honor the giver of that good gift is by stewarding the gift well.

I don't want to get carried away with the metaphor, but I'm sure you get where I'm going. When we view our bodies rightly and biblically as good gifts from God, given to us to fulfill our callings on this side of heaven, and understand that everything we have (including our bodies) is His, we are much more likely to care for our bodies appropriately, eschewing the extremes of idolatry and apathy. Not because we love or worship our bodies, but because we love and worship the One who gave them to us—the One who intelligently designed our bodies and created everything they would need—in the first place.

Friend, consider this book a formal invitation to get back to

God's design for us and live a little closer to how we were created to live—to do the slow, perhaps boring, everyday stewardship stuff while living in a society of speed, convenience, often confusing health advice, fads, and quick fixes—all from a place of obedience and freedom instead of obsession and fear.

Cozy up. This conversation is long overdue. I'm so glad I get to have it with you.

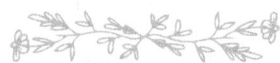

PRAYER

God, thank You for my body. Whether I am happy with where I am with my health or feel a long way off from where I'd like to be, help me to be a good steward of what You have given me. Help me treat my body as the good gift that it is instead of as a project to fix. I pray for discernment and wisdom in a world of many trends and opinions, and I pray that You would show me which steps are mine to take and which are not. Amen.

PRACTICAL APPLICATION

Take some time to reflect and ask yourself these questions from the chapter:

1. *Have I turned a good thing (such as my body or well-being) into a god thing?*
2. *Is it possible that a good intention has spiraled into obsession?*

3. *Am I ready to focus on living in alignment with God's design more than getting tangled up in all the world's health advice?*

Now prayerfully ask God to open your heart to receiving what He has to teach you and where He is leading you on your own unique health journey as you seek to be good to your body.

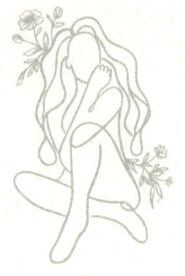

Chapter 2

WHERE ARE WE GOING WRONG?

I recently found a photo of my younger self, whom I described in the previous chapter, when I was at my leanest and at my lowest weight. It took me back to a time when I completely fell for all that's culturally "desirable" and what society says is healthy.

People would often ask me about my workouts, curious what I was doing to get in shape. And if you saw me, you might assume that because I was "in shape," I was super healthy.

While looking at the photo, I momentarily missed the shredded body of my past self and wondered if maybe I should try to get it back. But then I thought, *Mmm . . . better not.* At least, I better not in the way that I went about achieving it before.

Why? Because regardless of what I looked like on the outside, there was so much imbalance going on internally.

A few years after that photo was taken, I began a lot of testing to try to figure out what was going on inside my body. Through that, I found many eye-opening discoveries, such as that my adrenals were shot, my gut was a disaster, and my hormones were a mess.

Looking back, it makes sense as to why. Beyond working out and eating salads, the rest of my lifestyle was not all that healthy. I worked long hours and had no screen-time boundaries. I lived on multiple double-shot lattes a day and was basically dependent on coffee for energy (and I didn't even have kids then!). I skipped breakfast most days, didn't eat nearly enough protein, and used tons of products loaded with endocrine disruptors.

And it was only as I began to dig deeper that I learned health is so much more than fitness and green juice and that there was so much I didn't even realize was affecting my body.

ARE WE *WELL*?

For centuries, staying healthy was a means to an end—to survive, earn a living, raise a family, or accomplish a goal. This should still be the driving motivator for us today. We should be well enough to fulfill the callings on our lives, whether that looks like raising a family, working as an accountant or nurse, being a missionary, or fulfilling some other vocation.

However, for many, health has now become the end goal itself—to biohack and work our way to the perfect or optimal body. Health and the body have become idols that our world worships.

If you think about it, we have more health resources than ever before, from twenty-four-hour gyms to supplements and powders to online fitness coaches and diets galore. We have more information and tools than our ancestors could have ever imagined at our fingertips. We spend plenty of time and money on treatments, injections, prescriptions, and procedures. On top of that, doesn't it seem like there's always a new trend or hot new product hitting the market? Or is that just me?

Don't get me wrong. Some of these can be good and beneficial things.

But are we *well*? Are we *thriving*? In theory, with all these advancements and tools, we should be healthier than ever, right? But are we?

What is the research telling us about our health, specifically as women? The sources I've consulted show that despite medical and scientific advancements, women in the United States continue to experience health issues, and many of those health issues are still on the rise:

- Women account for 80 percent of people with autoimmune diseases, which are the third most prevalent disease category after cancer and heart disease.[1]
- Breast cancer diagnoses in women under age fifty have been increasing by more than 2 percent annually over the past five years and have increased steadily in women under age 50 over the past two decades.[2]
- Polycystic ovarian syndrome (PCOS) is the most common endocrine abnormality in women of reproductive age, and the prevalence of PCOS is increasing.[3]
- According to the American Thyroid Association (ATA), one in eight women will develop a thyroid disorder during their lifetimes, which is five to eight times more likely than for men.[4]
- Women are also disproportionately affected by chronic pain, depression, osteoporosis, and dementia. Female-

specific conditions like endometriosis are understudied and can often lack effective treatment options.[5]

With all the biohacking tools, 24/7 gyms, and information we have access to, you would think that society would be trending toward getting healthier, not sicker.

So what in tarnation is going on? Let's talk about it.

THE BIG C'S

Sometimes I feel as though society is trying to destroy women. I know saying that might be a little dramatic, but there's no denying that there's an endless barrage of health risks and harmful toxins everywhere we look and in everything we use and that women seem to have been hit hardest.

With all the toxin-laden cosmetics and implants, hormone-altering birth control, nutrient-deficient diets, and confusing "advice" thrown our way, it can be tough to be well. Some of this is being offered from people with good intentions, some by those with bad intentions (seeking profit or fame), and some purely out of ignorance.

Obviously, many things can influence our health, but if I had to choose a handful of key factors that I believe have influenced our bodies and well-being most, it would be the following *C*'s: convenience, cultural beauty standards, conflicting health advice, corporations and chemicals, and careers. Let's unpack those more.

Convenience

As a mom of two under two, I willfully admit I am thankful to have access to some conveniences. Grocery delivery? *Yes, please.* A ready-to-go smoothie pouch to give to my grumpy toddler when he's screaming in the back seat on a long road trip? *Basically manna from heaven.*

There are plenty of benefits to the conveniences available to us in today's world. But as with many good things, a culture of convenience doesn't come without a cost to our bodies.

According to PubMed, while advances in technology have provided many benefits to society, they have also led to a substantial reduction in the amount of incidental physical activity. Physical activities previously conducted as part of a "standard" working day (active transport, labor, and so on) or as part of domestic duties around the home (cleaning and cooking) have been reduced or replaced by machines.[6]

So now instead of living active lifestyles naturally, the majority of people live relatively sedentary lifestyles. If we want to be more active, we often sit in a car as we drive to a gym (that we pay for) to move our bodies and then sit in a car to drive home, picking up dinner-to-go on the way. We've accepted that as fine and normal, but I just don't think it's how we were meant to live.

Additionally, with the rise of convenience has come an increase in ultra-processed, prepackaged grab-and-go foods, or what some might call "food-like" products because of the amount of non-food ingredients in them. In fact, all the conveniences available to us have taken so many of us out of the kitchen. Instead of learning to cook or bake with real food, it's almost easier to turn to delivery or prepackaged microwave meals.

We are out of touch with our food—where it comes from and how it's prepared. We've sacrificed our connection to our food for the sake of convenience. We may have a lot to eat, but that doesn't necessarily mean we are well-nourished.

I was talking about this with my friend Annika, a functional nutritional therapy practitioner, and she said something that stood out to me: "As a society, we're eating more than ever but starving on a cellular level."

And now I can't unhear it.

Along those same lines, a large study found that "eating 10 percent more ultra-processed foods was associated with above a 10 percent increase in the risks of cardiovascular disease, coronary heart disease, and cerebrovascular disorders."[7]

So, are conveniences all bad? Should we avoid every snack and to-go food? Of course not. For one thing, there are many healthier handy options with better ingredients that we can seek out when possible. But I'd argue that it's a *dependence* on many of these conveniences that may not be serving us—or our health—well. And it may be wise to be mindful of how often we turn to these conveniences so as not to become reliant on them.

Cultural Beauty Standards

The pressure on us women to manipulate our bodies in the name of beauty is becoming unbearable. A quick scroll through social media tells us we need Botox injections, lip fillers, weight-loss medication, better body shapes, and more.

In fact, research from 2003 shows that girls develop a desire to be thinner starting at age six.[8] This research was conducted before the era of everyone having social media in their pockets, so I'd imagine that desire is even more prevalent now.

I'm all about presenting ourselves well, embracing our God-given beauty, and doing things that make us happy. I personally enjoy getting my nails done sometimes. But the pressure we can feel after checking out other people's social media is just too much. The things we have long been pressured to do at the expense of our long-term and short-term health just to keep up with a social-media-driven standard of beauty is out of control.

If that pressure has ever gotten to you, I don't blame you. I've felt it too.

There has to be a better, biblical way to care for our bodies and looks than all the artificial junk designed to manipulate our beauty to fit cultural beauty standards, right? *Right.* And that doesn't mean we should neglect beauty altogether. But maybe there's something we're missing. Maybe we could benefit from getting back to more natural treatments.

Conflicting Health Advice

Do you ever experience the frustration of finding some health information that seems to make sense, such as almond milk being healthier than whole milk, only to later stumble across something that directly contradicts it? You've been chugging almond milk for months, thinking you're doing a good thing, but then you come across another school of thought that leaves you second-guessing that decision entirely and wondering if perhaps you're missing key nutrients from dairy, and before you know it, you're back to square one. I mean, is almond milk healthy or not?

Okay, maybe that was just my experience. But that is why I started going back to the Bible and asking myself, *Did God create it?* to get clarity on those types of things. Of course, as with anything, there can still be nuance in how different individuals interpret these answers. One could argue that God gave us almonds, so therefore almond milk is healthy, while another could argue that, yes, He gave us nuts, but they are not made to be consumed in large amounts or in milk form, because nut milk is a man-made invention. Nevertheless, going back to the basics and asking, *What did God create, and how did He direct us to use that creation?* can help cut through some of the confusing opinions and information out there.

Moreover, I'd argue that it's possible that even health trends that are "research backed" aren't the ultimate truth and shouldn't be taken as gospel truth straightaway. Not only are the funding sources and possible conflicts of interest in said research something to consider, but I also recently learned that many studies for things such as popular diets may be primarily done on males, which can leave us women with many unanswered questions about what works for our divinely designed bodies (with a cycle).[9]

For example, let's look at a big trend that's taken off in recent years: intermittent fasting.

According to the Cleveland Clinic, intermittent fasting can actually have a negative effect on the female sex hormones progesterone and estrogen.[10] So it's not necessarily a quick and easy weight-loss fix for women, specifically for those of childbearing age or who are pre-menopausal. Throughout the menstrual cycle, estrogen and progesterone levels change. The rise and fall of hormones is chiefly regulated by gonadotropin-releasing hormone (GnRH).[11]

"GnRH can be very sensitive to environmental factors," registered dietitian Julia Zumpano states. "Things like fasting can keep it from doing its job and releasing the chemicals needed to stimulate estrogen and progesterone."[12]

So while we've heard all about the benefits and how amazing something like intermittent fasting is, many women are left feeling exhausted or worse than before they began the lifestyle and, understandably, confused as to why!

The point is that we get loads of information and come across a bunch of trendy health fads and bio hacks that may not even be biologically appropriate or beneficial for us. Much of the information might be from a study primarily done on men, and we just assume it can be copy/pasted to women. But women are *not* just smaller men.

Sifting through all the research, schools of thought, and fads is enough to make our heads spin. And, unfortunately, it can create a general apathy toward making healthy changes because it can feel impossible to do anything "right."

Therefore, we have to seek to understand and support our female physiology rather than just jumping on the next bandwagon the moment it pops up.

Corporations and Chemicals

Do corporations influence our bodies and well-being? Yes. For one thing, many companies capitalize on women's insecurities to sell them a product to "fix" something about their bodies or beauty, even if the solution they provide can make women sick or leave them worse off—whether the "fix" is Botox injections, toxic makeup, implants, birth control, weight-loss supplements, or low-calorie foods devoid of nutrients.

Why would they do that? Think about it. What is a corporation's primary goal? Profit. Maximum profit.

That can (and often does) lead to decisions to use the cheapest ingredients that are easy to mass-produce quickly in order to keep costs low and profits high. Know what it means for you and me? It means that *a lot* of potentially harmful ingredients—hormone disruptors, known carcinogens, allergens, additives—can end up in our everyday products and processed foods.

Not long ago, I came across a study that confirmed that girls are starting puberty earlier.[13] Another study concluded that exposure to phthalates may be associated with increased risk of early menstruation.[14] Phthalates and other hormone disruptors, such as parabens, have been in nearly every beauty, personal-care, and household-care product that women and girls have been using for decades.

As I uncovered these findings, it kind of all clicked for me. Personally, I started my period when I was just ten years old, and I was upset about it. My mom tried to celebrate my *passage to womanhood* with me, but it felt like a bad dream. I was just a kid! I wasn't ready to deal with those types of womanly things. Then, later in life, I was diagnosed with endometriosis. I also suffered recurrent pregnancy loss.

Not only that, but other studies have shown how much these toxic chemicals in everyday products can increase a woman's chances of getting diseases such as breast cancer. One study in particular saw a significant decrease in breast cancer cell gene expression when products with parabens and phthalates were removed for just twenty-eight days.[15]

While some of the worst offenders, like parabens, may be found in small amounts in a single product, when we consider all the products with these that we use or consume on a daily basis, our exposure can expand from tiny to enormous very quickly. (We'll talk more about that in chapter 7.)

The corporations make their money, we get sick, and then we we might turn to corporations (such as Big Pharma) for a solution to the problem they quite possibly had a hand in creating to begin with. Sounds pretty twisted when you step back and look at it through that lens, doesn't it?

Careers

Inherently, work is a good thing. Work is a gift from God. Genesis 2 tells us how He assigned Adam and Eve the job of taking care of His creation in the Garden of Eden. The work that God gave

Adam and Eve (and, in turn, us) was a gift He knew would bring them joy, connection, and purpose. He designed work to be a blessing to us and others, since doing meaningful work gives us a sense of fulfillment.

So why is "careers" on the list of things that influence our bodies and well-being? Because, like any good thing that's a gift from God, our broken world and sinful people can corrupt it.

And in many ways, it has been. Being "on" and available virtually anytime, thanks to the devices we carry in our pockets, together with the pressure to climb the corporate ladder and endure the nine-to-five grind, has turned us into a culture of overworked, burned-out people. It's not much better for entrepreneurs, either, as many would tell you they began a business to experience freedom and flexibility, only to find themselves working sixty or more hours per week just to keep the lights on.

Our bodies were not designed for this nonstop "slog." God designed our feminine physiology perfectly and creatively, with both circadian rhythms and infradian rhythms.

According to the National Institutes of Health (NIH), a *circadian rhythm* is the twenty-four-hour internal clock in our brains that regulates cycles of alertness and sleepiness by responding to light changes in our environment. Throughout the day, our hormones, organs, and bodily systems undergo several changes. From the time we wake up until the time we go to sleep, our internal clocks affect our moods, our ability to digest food, our internal temperatures, and many other physical, mental, and emotional processes.[16]

I interviewed Alisa Vitti, a hormone expert and researcher who teaches on feminine physiology, on my podcast a few times, and she taught me about these rhythms, namely the infradian rhythm, which I had never heard of before. It's fascinating!

An *infradian rhythm* is a biological cycle that occurs for longer than a twenty-four-hour period. A prime example of an infradian rhythm is the menstrual cycle. There are four phases to a menstrual cycle: follicular, ovulatory, luteal, and menstrual. Vitti teaches that during each of these four phases, you experience normal hormonal fluctuations that influence your body temperature, energy, emotions, and more. The twenty-eight-day cycle (infradian rhythm) works in close concert with a twenty-four-hour cycle, which means that a dysregulated infradian rhythm will mess with your circadian cycle, and a circadian cycle will negatively influence your infradian cycle. Here's how she explains it:

> People with female physiology benefit when they eat, exercise, and work in ways that support their infradian rhythm, as opposed to following diet, fitness, and work trends that disrupt it. It's precisely because so many women try to follow the "same-thing-everyday" plans that work for male physiology that 50% of women are suffering with hormonal imbalances, while men don't suffer them at the same rate.[17]

I could go on, but if you're interested in learning more on this, you can listen to the episode "Cycle Sync to Improve Productivity, Health, and Relationships" on my podcast that addresses the topic.[18]

When we don't honor those rhythms, our mental, physical, spiritual, and emotional health will inevitably be affected (as I know well from personal experience). And our society and the work culture that dominates our modern world aren't really set up to honor or support those very rhythms.

The early-morning wake-ups, the rigid schedule, a lack of boundaries, minimal flexibility, long commutes, stressful deadlines, late-night notifications, being so busy that we forget to eat lunch or we run out the door with an empty stomach and just a cup of coffee in the morning—all those make it nearly impossible to support our body's biological needs.

Obviously, not everyone can just quit their job. The point is that "the grind" and this culture obsessed with breaking glass ceilings and climbing the corporate or status ladder (or both) aren't helping us. And if you're feeling burned-out by it all, there's a good reason why. It's not because you're lazy; rather, it's because this lifestyle is not supportive to our very basic feminine biological needs.

I readily admit there was a time when I bought into the achievement culture. When I was younger, all I wanted was to attain big goals and dreams. But that mindset, and what I put my body through to get there, eventually affected my health, my hormones, and my fertility (even though I was sold the idea that I could "have it all"). I then made a conscious decision to shift my perspective (and my approach to work) tremendously.

Now my mindset says, *Forget glass ceilings and girl-bossing and give me slow mornings, time with my family, flexibility, and vitality,* even if that means I earn less, take longer to reach professional goals, or don't have society's status symbols of "success." Since that version of success burns me out and hurts my health, I don't want it. I like my own *healthy* version of success much better.

But our modern society is built around this crazy work schedule. We've been trained, and almost forced, to build our lives around work, as opposed to building work around our lives. Perhaps the best thing we can do is become aware of that fact and make simple shifts where possible to intentionally slow down, set boundaries, create rhythms of rest, and even consider work that is better suited to our needs, despite culture, higher education, and Instagram saying that means we're not "succeeding."

As I noted, these five factors—convenience, cultural beauty standards, conflicting health advice, corporations and chemicals, and careers—are far from a comprehensive list of wellness inhibitors, but they are major hurdles that can make it more difficult to live aligned with God's design. Does that mean we should all quit our jobs, never order groceries, make all our own products from scratch, and move off the grid? Of course not. I mean, that may sound nice, but it's not realistic for most of us.

But what if living a healthy life aligned with God's design didn't involve being afraid of all the "bad" stuff or running away from society (especially given that we're called to be a light *in* society)? What if it's as simple as revisiting what the Bible says, considering what we can modify in our modern lifestyle to be a little more aligned with God's design, and obediently making small shifts and doing the best we can right where we are?

I'D RATHER BE *WELL*

I spent years researching women's health, sifting through endless health advice from experts, and digging into approaches to healing online—which ultimately led to making a ton of changes to my lifestyle. I began slowing down, prioritizing my sleep, doing gentler workouts, making sure I was eating enough every day, restricting less, replenishing with bioavailable nutrients more, and gradually lowering my toxin burden.

Want to know what happened? My weight settled at about ten to fifteen pounds heavier than it was when I was chronically undereating. I didn't become overweight by gaining some weight; my body just settled where it naturally would when it was well fed and nourished instead of having critical nutrients and bioavailable fuel, like quality carbs, withheld. Interestingly, it settled right around where it was when I was in college, before I began aggressively exercising and obsessively counting calories in an effort to get extra lean.

So yeah, I'm not as lean as I once was, but I'm also metabolically and hormonally so much healthier than I have been in a long time. My skin cleared. My natural energy came back (until I had kids and quality sleep was harder to come by for a time, but that's a story for another day). My hormones balanced out a lot. My periods were no longer painful, and PMS symptoms virtually disappeared. And I not only got pregnant but also stayed pregnant and had a live baby for the first time in my life after recurrent pregnancy loss. I needed some medical support in pregnancy, too, such as blood thinners, but I truly believe that many of the lifestyle changes I made also helped support my fertility, body, and baby throughout pregnancy and postpartum recovery.

Typically, when we talk about getting healthy, the focus is on weight loss. And in many cases, that is part of the process. But my point is that health and healing is not a one-size-fits-all approach. Sometimes, allowing our bodies to find their natural weight when we begin to nourish them well *can* be healthier than running on stress hormones and undereating, intentionally or unintentionally.

And I don't know about you, but I don't want to be *just* super fit. I've been super fit while simultaneously being depleted nutritionally, which meant I was metabolically, hormonally, and emotionally unwell. That's not health—at least not holistically.

I'd rather be healthy holistically: physically, spiritually, mentally, and emotionally. Like the saying we slap on coffee mugs and stitch on pillows says, *It is well with my soul.*

I mean, if I hold a biblical view of the body—where the soul and body are not disconnected but are one—can it really be well with my soul if my body is starving or I'm running on stress hormones or overexercising?

So no, I don't want to be just *fit*; I also want to be *well*. And if that means I'm nourished and balanced and well rested but not as lean as humanly possible, that's okay with me.

I've had to do that all while giving myself a lot of grace along the way because all the conflicting health advice online and the way our society is set up really don't make it easy. But my goal simply became to be good (not perfect) to my body by getting a tiny bit closer to God's design, even if that's just 1 percent at a time.

> My goal simply became to be good to my body by getting a tiny bit closer to God's design, even if that's just 1 percent at a time.

And maybe if we focused less on manipulating, changing, forcing, and fixing our bodies and instead just started being good to them and giving them the good things God made, we might be able to be truly well in a world obsessed with fitness, filled with convenience and quick fixes, and littered with conflicting health advice.

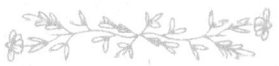

PRAYER

God, I want to partner with You in how I care for my body. Please show me where I can tend to my health better. Help me hear Your voice and use Your Word as my guide instead of getting caught up in all the voices and man-made ideas the world is throwing at me. I trust that You are above it all, that Your design is good, and that You have given me good things to support my body. Amen.

PRACTICAL APPLICATION

Which of the *C's*—convenience, cultural beauty standards, conflicting health advice, corporations and chemicals, and careers—may be taking the greatest toll on your body's well-being in this season of your life? Have you been relying on convenience or processed foods for most of your nourishment? Or maybe you've been hustling after professional goals, neglecting necessary rest, and relying on caffeine for energy?

Maybe it's something else entirely.

Consider which of those may be affecting your health the most and decide on a few specific adjustments you can make. For example, if you have been relying on convenience, like delivery and prepackaged processed foods for most meals, perhaps you can commit to cooking dinner at home four to six nights a week for the next three months.

Prayerfully decide what changes you will make to be good to your body in light of the five common obstacles to your being well.

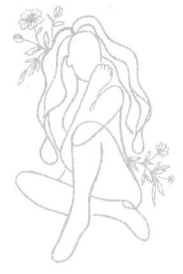

Chapter 3

WHAT DOES THE BIBLE SAY?

Shortly after my son was born, I was rocking him in his room and looked to the banner hanging on his wall. The words "fearfully and wonderfully made" (from Psalm 139:14) are printed on it. I'd read that passage a thousand times, but for some reason, on that day in particular, the word *fearfully* stood out to me.

Fearfully? Wait, why does it say "fearfully"? I wondered. *What does that word mean? Scared?*

So while my newborn napped on my chest, I grabbed my phone and looked it up.

I learned that the word *fearfully* in Hebrew is *yare,* which means "reverence" or "respect."[1] As it's translated, *fearfully* isn't about being *scared;* rather, it's about being in the presence of something *sacred.* As author Lori Stanley Roeleveld says, "This type of 'fear' is like the sense of awe or astonishment that overcomes us in a magnificent cathedral, staring out over a great range of mountains at sunrise or when holding a newborn."[2] It's wonder, amazement, awe, and reverence. Just like I feel when I look at my children, that is how our Father sees us as His creation and His children: sacred.

So, if our bodies are fearfully and wonderfully made, if they are sacred to their creator, it only makes sense to treat them with reverence and respect, right?

Treating our bodies with the kind of reverence and respect they were designed for is so much deeper than the body-positive language and empty self-love affirmations that society offers. First, it requires a right view of the body—that it is a sacred vessel to carry out our callings. I've already mentioned this, but it bears repeating: Our bodies were made to worship and glorify *God*, not to *be* "gods" we obsess over.

> Our bodies were made to worship and glorify *God*, not to *be* "gods" we obsess over.

And it is a holy pursuit to holistically care for the bodies we've been given—to nourish, move, rest, and give our bodies the good things God designed for them to thrive.

Treating our bodies with reverence and respect begins with understanding that they are sacred, considering the biblical guidelines for wellness that God laid out from the beginning of time, and taking steps to live aligned with our creator's design.

SO, WHAT IS GOD'S DESIGN?

In His Word, God has provided fundamental principles to guide our choices in ways that promote health and well-being. For example, Genesis tells us that God rested from His work on the seventh day of creation (see 2:2). Since we are made in His image, that means *we* are designed to rest too—and not rest randomly but instead rhythmically and regularly.

Additionally, we are designed to eat what our creator gave us for nourishment: simple, wholesome food from the earth, not man- or lab-made, chemical-laden, heavily processed items packaged and sold as "food." God said, "I give you every seed-bearing plant on the face of the whole earth and every tree that has fruit with seed in it. They will be yours for food.... Everything that lives and moves about will be food for you. Just as I gave you the green plants, I now give you everything" (1:29; 9:3, NIV).

Now, this nourishment may have been easier for our ancestors because food in Bible times was more wholesome and void of harmful chemicals. People ate food according to God's design. There weren't heavily processed, lab-made, and chemical-laden foods back then.

Despite being fundamentally very simple, eating healthier food requires more effort nowadays. Why? Because we likely have to go out of our way to source quality food that is in its most natural or whole form—in other words, food that is closest to how God designed it before it was corrupted by humans trying to do it better, easier, and faster (and, quite frankly, cheaper). These days, processed, mass-produced, and convenient food is much easier to come by. In fact, it's more accessible and often considered more affordable since it can be produced quickly and cheaply in large quantities, often with the addition of pesticides, herbicides, and even preservatives to make it last longer.

Some might say it's high-maintenance to prioritize sourcing quality food (that which is whole and unadulterated). And while healthy eating can absolutely become an unhealthy obsession (a conversation for a later chapter), I can't help but think of the virtuous woman in Proverbs 31 and how she gathered and obtained food for her family. Verse 14 describes her like this: "She is like the ships of the merchant; she brings her food from afar." That is, she went out of her way to find the best for her family. She does not settle for what is convenient—she seeks what is good.

How applicable to our modern life! Sometimes what's convenient isn't what's best, and it's not bougie or high-maintenance to seek out the best for our bodies and families within our means. According to the Bible, it's actually virtuous. I don't know about you, but I want to live as virtuously as possible, even if that means going out of my way to source real food and better-quality products that help me live more aligned with God's design.

As I dig into the Bible, I find that living aligned with His design is quite simple. It's not the latest fad diet or newest weight-loss trend or the fanciest workout plan. It's literally just being as intentional as possible to give our bodies the good things He created (in the form closest to how He created them).

Rest regularly. Eat real food. Spend time in nature, in God's creation. Move your body. Although doing all that sounds simple, information overload and endless health trends can make it seem more difficult than it needs to be.

Is it possible that part of the reason so many of us are sick and stressed-out is that some of the health advice we've listened to is unbiblical and is basically backward? That we've gotten so incredibly far away from nature and what God designed for our bodies that we've complicated things?

How we care for our bodies and how we feel physically directly affects our mental, spiritual, and emotional health. God is clear that He cares about our health, and therefore so should we. The biblical principles of health are important, reasonable, and practical, and countless verses in the Bible are devoted to the subject. So when the next wave of wellness trends swells, when we come across conflicting health advice or feel as though we can't keep up or do anything right, we must go back to the fundamentals:

- What did God create in the first place?
- What guidelines does the Bible give for being good to our bodies?
- How can we live even 1 to 2 percent closer to God's design?

When I looked to the Bible for those answers, I uncovered foundational truths and simple guidelines that can serve as an anchor, or guide, as we aim to be good stewards of our bodies (and be good examples in society) when fear or confusion (or both) begins to rise.

> Supporting your body's ability to heal and thrive looks like giving it the good things God created—not fixing, forcing, or punishing it by overworking it, using diet pills, restricting food, or subjecting it to invasive procedures to manipulate its appearance.

PRINCIPLES FOR BEING GOOD TO YOUR BODY

Supporting your body's ability to heal and thrive looks like giving it the good things God created—not fixing, forcing, or punishing it by overworking it, using diet pills, restricting food, or subjecting it to unnecessary invasive procedures to manipulate its appearance.

If I had to summarize what I found in Scripture, I'd say that, ultimately, being good to your body means glorifying God with it. But what does that look like practically? Let's start in Genesis—in the beginning—when God made human bodies and created everything they needed to thrive. According to what I found in the Bible, being good to your body looks like the following principles.

1. Honor Your Femininity and Biological Needs

Genesis 1:27 says, "God created man in his own image, in the image of God he created him; male and female he created them."

We are made in the image of God, and our creator made male and female differently. This fact alone should influence the way we work, eat, move, and live. As we've noted already, women are not just mini men; we are created uniquely, with specific biological needs. The way we work and rest, how we exercise, and the nourishment we need should ultimately support our divinely designed bodies and feminine physiology. Being good to our bodies involves celebrating our femininity and distinct biological needs instead of trying to be like men or keep up with hustle culture (which is quite masculine). Our society may tell us that approach is weak or sexist, but I'm willing to bet the One who created all things, including male and female biology, has a little more wisdom than ever-changing cultural norms. So I don't know about you, but I'm going to go with Him as my guide.

2. Cultivate a Healthy Environment

Genesis 1:28 says, "God blessed them. And God said to them, 'Be fruitful and multiply and fill the earth and subdue it, and have dominion over the fish of the sea and over the birds of the heavens and over every living thing that moves on the earth.'"

God blessed humankind, and part of that blessing was to "be fruitful." He also gave us dominion over the earth. What does that mean for us as we aim to be good to our bodies?

First, being given dominion over the earth and creation does not mean we can abuse them. Instead, we have been tasked with being good stewards—to care for and nurture the world around us. When we consider the fact that our bodies not only are part of creation but also depend on creation to survive, we see that being good to our bodies is obediently following this command. It is cultivating a healthy environment, one that supports both our individual and our collective well-being.

That includes creating an environment and lifestyle that supports our fertility (instead of suppressing it with toxic chemicals). That's not to say we all need to have babies to be good to our bodies, and it's also not to say we'll avoid any struggle with infertility if we don't intentionally suppress it. But it does mean doing what we can to create an environment both within and around our bodies that *supports* our hormones and fertility. That may look like reducing our toxin exposure where we can, swapping plastic for glass when possible, getting a few houseplants or using an air purifier, or keeping our living environment clean and healthy.

All of that said, it's imperative to emphasize that being fruitful is so much more than having babies. While God may call humanity to be fruitful in the sense of populating the earth, what I'm ultimately getting at is that this verse from Genesis reminds us that we are to be fruitful in all areas of life. Cultivating a fruitful environment in which to live—one that is peaceful and healthy—allows us to feel our best and be fruitful in the work we do, conversations we have, and ways that we spend our time, talents, and resources. This is a high calling. Perhaps being fruitful in this season looks like creating something beautiful, serving in a ministry, cooking healthy food for your family, donating to those in need, starting a neighborhood garden, decluttering areas in your home, or leading a Bible study. It could be a combination of a few of those or something else not listed here.

Fruitfulness means, in essence, contributing to the flourishing of humankind, and that begins with the flourishing of our own bodies and our own families. It's bringing heaven to earth—using our gifts, skills, and talents to make the space around us a little more Eden-like.

Think about it: How can we be fruitful if we're burned-out, overworked, dealing with imbalance, or feeling terrible? Or if we're undernourished, sleeping poorly, low on energy, or running on stress hormones?

It's so much harder.

While it may be *normal* to skip breakfast, stay up late scrolling, order carryout for most meals, or use products with harmful chemicals or hormonal birth control to suppress our unwanted symptoms (or fertility), that does not make these common practices *good* for our bodies, as those actions do not support fruitfulness. This command, or calling, to be fruitful and multiply the kingdom of God reminds us that being good to our bodies—caring for ourselves and supporting our health naturally with our daily choices and disciplines—requires being thoughtful about and cultivating a healthy environment for them to live in.

Doing so is critical to fulfilling our God-given callings, whether that calling looks like raising a family, leading a Bible study, serving the needy, or something else entirely.

3. Nourish Your Body with Real Food

Genesis 1:29 reads, "God said, 'Behold, I have given you every plant yielding seed that is on the face of all the earth, and every tree with seed in its fruit. You shall have them for food.'" And Genesis 9:3 says, "Every moving thing that lives shall be food for you. And as I gave you the green plants, I give you everything."

Is it just me, or does it feel as though food—and what makes a food healthy—is hotly debated? I mean, are nut milks and nut flours healthy or harmful? Should we drink cow's milk? Eat animal protein? Cruciferous vegetables? It literally can depend on whom you ask. And it's all a little confusing, isn't it?

Some might argue that based on the Creation account, humans should need to eat only vegetation, or plants, to survive. But the truth is that based on Genesis 9, after the fall of man, God gave all living creatures—plants *and* animals—to be food for us. And Jesus ate meat, so there's that, too.

Although humans may have originally needed to eat only plants, being permitted to eat both plants and animals is a result of the Fall. And the fact is, we live in a post-Fall world. And perhaps God, in His wisdom, may have known that we—who would no longer live in the garden full of unadulterated, perfectly nourishing plants—may also need animal products to thrive, so He permitted both.

While we could debate specifics like these all day, I think what's most important to understand is that being good to our bodies entails nourishing them with what God made and directed us to eat.

4. Slow Down and Rest Regularly

The Creation account alone clearly reveals that we are made to rest. God intentionally separated night and day, as if to say, "This is the rhythm in which you are designed to work, rest, and play."

Genesis 1:5 says, "God called the light Day, and the darkness he called Night. And there was evening and there was morning, the first day." Then in verse 14, God said, "Let there be lights in the expanse of the heavens to separate the day from the night. And let them be for signs and for seasons, and for days and years."

This tells us we have a divinely designed biological clock that is built to be in sync with the natural light God made. While the lightbulb and iPhone are incredible advancements that have come with many blessings (thank you, Thomas Edison and Steve Jobs), the downside is that all the artificial light and screens we have access to daily can so easily disrupt this God-designed system known as the circadian rhythm.

Does that mean we should never have a light on after the sun goes down? Of course not. Especially in the winter, when in many places, like the Midwest, the sun goes down before 5:00 P.M. Yes, it's brutal.

It *does* mean that being good to our bodies requires us to support our circadian rhythms and biological needs, such as by setting boundaries on screens and prioritizing quality sleep. Plus, Genesis 2 tells us that God Himself rested: "On the seventh day God finished his work that he had done, and he rested on the seventh day from all his work that he had done" (verse 2).

If we look at Jesus's life in the Gospels, we see that He also retreated and rested. If we are made in God's image (we are), and God Himself, who is limitless, rested, then how much more do we, who are limited, need rest?

He gave us the example of how to live, both through His creation *of* the earth and His time as a man *on* the earth. Our creator rested when He *created* humans and when He *became* a human. That tells me that being good to our bodies requires resting—regularly and rhythmically.

5. Move and Spend Time in Nature

Genesis 2:15 says, "The LORD God took the man and put him in the garden of Eden to work it and keep it." Do you want to know what I find especially interesting about this single sentence in the Creation account—from when humans were *first* created? God could have put them literally anywhere. He could have created a city or an office building or anything. I mean, He's God, right? He didn't need to wait for men to figure out how to make those structures. But He placed the very first human being in a garden. A *garden*! Not a concrete jungle with lots of sounds or a cubicle with stale coffee and fluorescent lighting, but a garden. In nature.

This single verse also highlights that God didn't place humans in the garden to just sit around. He placed them there for a purpose: to work it and keep it. That tells me the human body was designed to *move*—that we're supposed to be active—and to be in nature. It reveals our need for fresh air, sunlight, meaningful work, and purposeful exercise.

Modern science only confirms what the Bible has told us all along. A 2018 study observed the health benefits of being outdoors and found that increased outdoor exposure was associated with various health benefits, such as decreased cortisol and decreased diastolic blood pressure, as well as decreased risk of preterm birth, type 2 diabetes, and cardiovascular death.[3]

6. Be in Community

When we think of health, vegetables and exercise are generally some of the first things to come to mind. But you know what else is a key element to well-being, at least according to the Bible? Community.

Genesis 2:18 says, "It is not good that the man should be alone; I will make him a helper fit for him." The creator of our bodies quite literally said that it is *not* good to be alone, so He created a *good* solution to that problem: another person to be in relationship with.

We are relational beings because God is three in one: Father, Son, and Holy Spirit. His very being is relational. And as I already stated, we are made in His image. Plus, if we look at Jesus in the Gospels, we see how much He prioritized community and relationships. He walked with His followers. He broke bread with His friends. His mission, the entire purpose for which He came, was centered on the premise of mending the relationship between humans and the Father for eternity—a relationship that sin severed.

Our God is deeply relational, and therefore so are we.

If being good to our bodies means glorifying God, and we do that by giving our bodies the good things God made for them, wouldn't you agree that being in community and having healthy relationships is one way to care for our well-being? Our physical health is inseparable from our emotional, mental, and spiritual health. They holistically work together.

I could be as fit and hormonally balanced as possible but still feel terrible if I'm lonely or full of anxiety, right? Isolation does not support our health. While we all crave deep, meaningful, like-minded friendships, I'm keenly aware of the fact that those can be hard to find during some seasons of life. But even if we haven't yet found our besties in our current season or location, we can still be involved in our local community in many different ways: by supporting local farmers, knowing our neighbors, joining a book club or nearby gym, or plugging into a local church.

Whatever it looks like, being involved in a community is a critical component we cannot overlook when it comes to stewarding our health and well-being.

7. Live Life Fully

In Genesis 3, we see the fall of humanity:

> The serpent said to the woman, "You will not surely die. For God knows that when you eat of it your eyes will be opened, and you will be like God, knowing good and evil." So when the woman saw that the tree was good for food, and that it was a delight to the eyes, and that the tree was to be desired

to make one wise, she took of its fruit and ate, and she also gave some to her husband who was with her, and he ate. Then the eyes of both were opened, and they knew that they were naked. (verses 4–7)

What is *that* about? Why is it relevant to this conversation?

It's relevant because the world we live in is fallen and marred by sin, which means we will experience brokenness. We could live a perfectly healthy lifestyle and we still won't escape death or decay.

While it is wise to be informed about how to best care for our bodies, if what's ultimately driving our decisions is *fear* (of death, illness, infertility, and so on), healthy habits will quickly become idols and we will be stressed-out, miserable, and far from God. Instead of worshipping God by caring for creation (in this case, our bodies), we begin to worship the creation itself.

Aiming for utopia in a broken world only leads to a dystopian life.

Instead of glorifying God, we glorify ourselves. Instead of obeying God, we want to be our own god. We crave wisdom and control, like Eve did. And in the words of my friend Mal, we so long for Eden that sometimes, in our vicious pursuit of replicating it, we obsess over trying to control every single thing. As a result, we do what destroyed Eden in the first place. (I know from personal experience.)

So, as we seek to be good stewards of our bodies, it is absolutely critical to understand that we will not achieve perfection on earth. We will not re-create Eden here. Any delusion that we have of avoiding all risk or suffering will quickly go from obediently caring for creation into obsessively trying to control it. Aiming for utopia in a broken world only leads to a dystopian life, which may be marked by things like idolatry and disordered eating.

Treating healthy living as a means to an end (obediently caring for our bodies in the ways we are able so we can carry out our callings for the glory of God) and not as an end (or god) itself can help us keep a healthy heart posture in this. Being good to our bodies isn't just avoiding "bad" things or biohacking our way through our days; it's also enjoying the gift of life! As Proverbs 17:22 reminds us, "a cheerful heart is good medicine" (NIV). In other words, joy is literally good for your health.

> Pursuing true health doesn't mean keeping up with the newest biohacking trends, the latest fad diets, or fancy supplements; it means simply getting back to the basics of what God created for us.

You can drink green juice and lift weights and do all the healthy things in the world, but if your spirit is crushed under the weight of stress, control, and perfectionism? That will take a toll on your health. It just will. Even the Bible says so.

So while being good to your body often looks like eating whole foods, avoiding toxic chemicals, and exercising, sometimes it can *also* look like going to your favorite local hole-in-the-wall restaurant and laughing your butt off with your best friends over a delicious meal *without* stressing about the calories (or dare I say, *seed oils*).

WHAT DOES ALL THIS MEAN?

Our bodies live in a broken world. We won't experience total wholeness on this side of heaven, so our bodies need to be supported, not fixed.

The best way to support our bodies—to steward and be good to them instead of trying to fix or punish them—is to live in alignment with those seven biblical principles as much as possible. We need to seek out and give our bodies more of the good things God created for them—such as rest, real food, intentional movement, fresh air, and sunlight—and less of the man-made junk that surrounds us.

Pursuing true health doesn't mean keeping up with the newest biohacking trends, the latest fad diets, or fancy supplements; it means simply getting back to the basics of what God created for us. It's living a little more naturally in a world of synthetic and processed everything. It means seeking replenishing nutrients in a world of restrictive diets. It's getting more sunlight and less blue light. It's fearing God instead of fearing the future. I'm sure you get where I'm going with this. Needless to say, the list could go on.

Although we live in a broken world riddled with decay and disease, let's not forget that our bodies are God-given blessings and are worthy of good things.

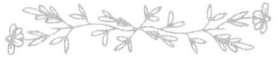

PRAYER

God, when I feel overwhelmed or confused by all the conflicting health advice in the world around me, help me come back to Your Word and focus on the basics of what You created: foundational guidelines to support my body. And when I begin to criticize my body or overwork it in order to achieve the results I think I desire instead of giving my body the rest it needs, help me remember that You say I am fearfully and wonderfully made, in Your image. You say that my body is sacred and a blessing, given to me to carry out the calling You put on my life—to be fruitful and multiply Your kingdom—and that it is worthy of good things, from real food to fun and relationships to rest. Thank You for those gifts. Amen.

PRACTICAL APPLICATION

What is one change you can make to better support your biological needs? Consider choosing one of the following activities to concentrate on every day for two weeks and see if you notice any differences:

- *Create rhythms of rest.*
- *Eat more whole, nourishing foods.*
- *Spend time in nature (fresh air, sunshine, ground beneath your feet).*
- *Invest in building community and relationships.*
- *Move your body.*
- *Cultivate a healthier living environment (reduce toxins, get rid of clutter, etc.).*
- *Live life fully by incorporating more joy and wholesome fun into your life.*

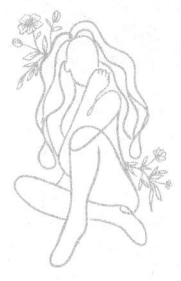

Chapter 4

WHY DOES BEING GOOD
TO YOUR BODY MATTER?

It was 2020 when I began learning more about our toxic and seemingly unsafe current environment, whether poor-quality soil, problems with conventional farming practices, too much exposure to electromagnetic fields (EMFs) from Wi-Fi and devices, or harmful ingredients in most packaged food as well as everyday products sold on shelves. And one day as I was walking through the grocery store, I caught myself vacillating between moments of panic that almost everything seemed unhealthy for me and moments of absolute apathy toward that reality.

One moment while shopping, I stopped to read a food label, saw all the fake ingredients in it, and became angry. The more I became aware of all the potential risks around me, the more it seemed as if everything was somehow trying to harm me. *Ugh, everything is going to kill me!* I thought in frustration as I put the item back on the shelf.

A few minutes later, I read another label with not-so-great ingredients and, feeling hopeless, tossed the item into my cart while thinking, *Whatever. Everything's going to kill me anyway. Might as well enjoy* something.

I felt like a crazy person! It was as though I couldn't decide if I wanted to be angry or apathetic at the fact that it seemed that my health was up against so many obstacles in our modern society.

Have you ever felt that way? Some days you want to do all you can to make the best choices for your body, and other days it just feels like too much and it's tempting to just ignore it all completely?

I'm with you, so let's talk about it.

IS EVERYTHING GOING TO KILL ME?

There's an old adage people tend to say when presented with health information: "Everything will kill ya!" It sounds kind of gloom and doom, doesn't it? But is it true?

In some ways, yes, it *is* true. We live in a fallen world and we can't escape death. Last I checked, the death rate is 100 percent, so to some extent, yes, everything *will* kill you. Eventually.

Diseases, physical hazards, mental health issues, accidents, the food you eat, the air you breathe, the water you drink, the toxins you're exposed to, sugar . . . Practically everything that exists in the world is actively working toward your death over the long-term, and many things are acutely dangerous, to some degree, over the short-term.

From a biblical perspective, there was only one time in the history of the world that people were without sin and the consequence of that sin. That time was in Genesis 2, when Adam and Eve were in the Garden of Eden, before sin messed everything up for all of us. Then, in Genesis 3, things changed. Eve craved wisdom, knowledge, and I'd even say control.

The subtle lie whispered by the serpent—that God didn't have Eve's best interests in mind and therefore must be withholding good things from her when He said not to eat from a certain tree—led her to want to be the one to decide what was best for her. She wanted to be in charge of her own destiny.

And how did that turn out for her (and all of humanity)? Well, it caused her to sin against God and, through that, opened all of us up to a world that is touched by the consequences of sin.

So, what does that mean for you and me?

Because we exist in a fallen world, toxic ingredients, unhealthy environments, and broken bodies *will* exist as well. We will all be touched by disease and decay in some way and all die eventually, no matter how much bone broth we drink or how many workouts we do.

We're not all that different from Eve. We crave wisdom and control, like she did. And we long for a world that isn't broken and where our bodies aren't touched or marred by disease, decay, and death. We long for Eden—for harmony, optimal health, perfection—so much that we may obsess over and try to control every single thing in our vicious pursuit of replicating it.

And as a result, we can easily put controlling creation over trusting the Creator.

Try as we may, we cannot replicate Eden. And the hard truth is that even the best things on earth won't come close to being as good or healthy or beautiful as heaven's worst. Does that mean we just shouldn't pay attention to what we use, do, or eat? Since it really doesn't change the fact that we will eventually die anyway? Is it an absolute waste to even bother with trying to give our bodies good things? We can't fix everything, so does that mean we shouldn't *do* anything?

Absolutely not. The fact that we can't escape decay or death is no excuse to just throw in the towel and do whatever we want; it's just a gut check when we start to spiral into the broken belief that we are in charge and can control everything.

Interestingly, I've noticed the "Everything's gonna kill ya" phrase is often said or used in one of two ways: It's either a deeply feared reality that leads us to stress out about anything that may be unhealthy, or it's an excuse for apathy, where we essentially do nothing to be better stewards of our bodies. Have you ever acted either of those ways? Or even straddled the tension of feeling both ways, perhaps at the same time?

Think about how I felt at the grocery store: One minute the reality that everything's going to kill us made me angry and led me to believe I needed to control every little thing. The next minute, it discouraged me and led me to believe the lie that the choices I make really don't matter at all.

Both are wrong responses.

So what's the *right* response?

Stewardship.

And that may go something like this: "True, I can't escape death and will be touched by brokenness on this side of heaven. But everything I have is Yours, God. I will be faithful in caring for my health so that I can fulfill the calling on my life well."

WHY STEWARDSHIP?

I truly believe that the church has failed to fulfill our call to steward our health well. Oh sure, we'll talk about it. We use the word *stewardship*, although many of us could hardly define it accurately. But if we were truly living out what we say we believe (that God gave us instructions for how to care for our bodies, cares about our health and well-being, and made the proper fuel we need), we would be setting the standard for healthy living and being good to our bodies. The world would be looking to us instead of the other way around.

For far too long, we have been guilty of following society when we should be leading the way. We so easily get tangled up in the cultural norms even if they're absolutely terrible for our bodies and we're quick to jump on the latest health trends. No wonder we're confused to no end. When we listen to other voices more than God's and follow health gurus more than we follow His guidelines, it will always feel like we're facing conflicting advice. *Because we are.*

But in Scripture, God provides fundamental principles to guide our personal choices in ways that promote health and prevent disease. And you know what's absolutely fascinating to me? As I researched this topic, I learned that in ancient Israel, it actually was the job of the priests—not physicians or health gurus—to provide basic health instruction and oversee the wellness of God's people. For example, in Leviticus 13, we learn that the priest was responsible for diagnosing leprosy and distinguishing it from other diseases.

Isn't that so interesting?

While nowadays we'd probably rather choose a doctor or similar expert when it comes to medical issues, I do think there's a lesson in that: As God's people, *we* should be setting the example and the standard for society on what it looks like to care for our health. I think if we took that responsibility seriously, we would be so much more likely to remain grounded and consistent in how we care for our health, even when everyone around us is jumping on bandwagons or even falling into the ever-so-easy trap of neglecting their health almost entirely.

I mentioned earlier that there have been times I've obsessed over healthy living because I was overcome by fear. However, there have *also* been times I've just followed culture's leading: I've overworked myself, consumed way too much caffeine, stayed up too late scrolling, jumped on fad diets, ordered takeout more than I cooked nourishing meals, and been so busy that I failed to eat breakfast. Instead of being a good steward of my body, I settled for what was normal in society (hustle, chronic busyness, convenience).

Want to know what happened?

Not surprisingly, I felt terrible. I had very little energy. I was impatient and moody. I had hormonal imbalances and painful periods. I snapped at my husband more easily. And ultimately, I really wasn't doing a very good job of serving God or showing up for the important work He put in front of me.

> What we do today directly affects our bodies tomorrow.

So while it's absolutely possible for wellness to become an obsession, I'd argue that being good to our bodies isn't just a trendy catch phrase; it's an act of obedience.

Remember, when we were formed out of the dust, our creator commanded us to care for and have dominion over creation (including our bodies). It's our job to obey that command and live aligned with His guidelines.

BEING GOOD TO OUR BODIES MATTERS IN ETERNITY

I know social media can make wellness things like low-tox swaps, organic recipes, fitness routines, and biohacking seem extra, unnecessary, or trendy.

And they *can* be.

But it's equally true that what we do today directly affects our bodies tomorrow. And how we care for our physical bodies and how well we feel directly affects our mood and energy, our families, our fertility, and, ultimately, how well we fulfill our God-given callings.

Investing in our well-being is an investment into eternity. We can't afford to neglect it. It is so integrally connected to our legacy. So no, we will never be able to care for our bodies 100 percent perfectly, and we won't even be able to do it well until we accept that reality (that's why this book is not called *Be Perfect to Your Body*). However, being thoughtful about the choices we make and how we invest into our well-being isn't trendy, vain, or worldly.

Being *good* to your body matters—not just now but also in light of eternity.

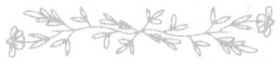

PRAYER

God, I trust that You have the answers I need. Help me keep my eyes fixed on You and Your statutes instead of getting tangled up in trends or tossed to and fro by the ever-changing cultural norms in modern society. I ask for the wisdom and discernment to see through what is confusing, be an example of what it looks like to be a good steward of the body You gave me, and come back to the timeless disciplines and guidelines that will help me be healthy. From this point forward, I commit to holding Your voice above all others, viewing every new trend I come across in the world around me through the lens of Scripture, and obeying Your Word when it comes to how I care for my body. Amen.

PRACTICAL APPLICATION

Make one positive change to support your body just a little better today. I'm not talking about jumping on the next trend or panicking over the latest study. Just make one small, better decision today. Maybe that looks like cooking a nutrient-rich dinner at home, going for a thirty-minute walk after lunch, or choosing to read instead of scroll before bed. Just one thing—one thing you can realistically do today and ideally repeat again tomorrow and the next day and the next, until it becomes a habit. One small change at a time adds up. And remember, what you do today directly affects your body tomorrow.

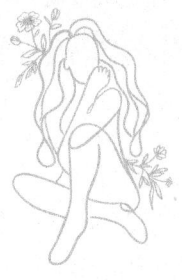

Chapter 5

REFRAME YOUR BODY BELIEFS

I was pee-my-pants nervous as I walked into the surgery center for a diagnostic laparoscopy and hysteroscopy in hopes of finding answers to my fertility challenges. Between miscarriages, gnarly PMS symptoms, and suddenly being unable to get pregnant altogether (although conception had been relatively quick and easy the first couple of times), I was feeling angry at my body. I felt as though it had failed me.

I'd been poked and prodded for endless tests already. The thought of willingly lying on an operating table to be cut open and investigated made me feel vulnerable, like I was a failure as a woman.

I was nervous that the doctors would find something (like endometriosis) and what that could mean. And I was equally nervous they wouldn't find anything, leaving me with nothing more than a scar and no further clarity than I had before.

Have you ever felt like that? Like your body is failing you? Maybe because of infertility, or maybe because of something else, such as hair loss, skin issues, or a chronic illness?

Whatever it is, if there's something that's causing you disappointment in and a little bit (or a lot) of frustration toward your body, I want to talk about it, because I know from personal experience that when I believed my body was failing me, I looked at it like it was a science project or experiment to figure out more than as a blessing. I spent more time criticizing it than caring for it. I resented it, and, as a result, I tried to manipulate and control it by doing things like restricting major food groups more than I replenished minerals and nutrients.

It's hard to give your body good things when you do not believe it *is* a good thing.

And the truth is, it's really difficult to be good to your body when you're believing lies about it. It's not natural to care for your body when you're constantly criticizing or trying to correct it. It's hard to give your body good things when you do not believe it *is* a good thing. It's tough to replenish your body with the nutrients or rest that it needs when you literally resent it.

When you believe that your body has failed you, pursuing health can quickly feel like a project or a punishment rather than a privilege. So in order to be good stewards of the bodies we've been given, we have to address the beliefs we have about them and filter those beliefs through the lens of what the Bible says about them.

WHAT IF YOUR BODY *ISN'T* FAILING YOU?

I groggily awoke from the surgery to see my husband with an eager look on his face.

"What'd they say?" I asked as I closed my eyes to shield them from the lights of the recovery room.

"They found endometritis *and* endometriosis!" he said excitedly, clearly grateful for answers.

I wasn't sure I was as excited. On the one hand, answers—that's good, right? But on the other hand, a low-grade chronic infection in my uterine lining (endometritis) *and* chronic disease in my body (endometriosis)? That's not exactly a good thing.

I sat there quietly for a moment, processing it all.

It's weird: When you spend years battling with your body, it's almost like you want "bad" news. You want a clear diagnosis and answer so you can finally address the problem at hand. In a way, that kind of clarity helps you have more compassion toward your body. Otherwise, it just seems like it is being a big jerk for no apparent reason.

Wow, I thought. *I've been over here being mad at my body for failing me, and this whole time it's been fighting a nasty disease and an infection. I had no idea.*

Did you catch that? I thought my body was *failing* me, when in reality it was *fighting* for me. But it took clarity for me to be able to see and believe that.

Unfortunately, we don't always get the clarity. We don't always know exactly what is going on, or it can take years to find out. I mean, in the case of endometriosis, it typically takes about a decade to get a diagnosis. *A decade.*[1]

That means the average woman with just this specific disease may spend ten years (or more) of her life believing the lie that her body is broken or failing. In reality, it is just doing its dang best with what it has to work with to fight for her every day.

My body and your body aren't defective or don't work improperly for no reason. Our bodies aren't failing us; they are fighting for us in a fallen world that fails us. As we long for the restoration and wait for the wholeness of heaven, our bodies exist outside the garden. Every single day, they're up against obstacles that inhibit their ability to thrive, from environmental toxins to highly stressful situations and everything in between. And although I've said it before, this feels like an appropriate place to say it again: In one way or another, every single one of us *will* be touched by death, decay, and disease.

Our bodies aren't failing us; they are fighting for us in a fallen world that fails us.

So whether or not you have a specific answer or diagnosis, and whether it's pain, infertility, acne, or some other symptom that's making you feel as though your body is failing, I want to encourage you to ask yourself this question: *What if my body isn't failing me but instead is fighting for me?*

It's not your body's fault. It's sin's fault—it's the result of the Fall. And your body isn't broken. It was designed with the brilliance and glory of heaven. But it *does* live in a fallen world, and that means it will be touched by brokenness.

Just some food for thought.

CARE MORE THAN YOU CRITICIZE

Has your internal monologue about your body ever sounded something like this: "Ugh, what is wrong with me?" or "I need to cover up my cellulite," or "Man, I wish I had [insert desired trait or different feature here]!"? Mine has. Whether I have been frustrated about acne, infertility, cellulite, or something else, I know I have been guilty of wasting way too much time and energy criticizing my body.

But as I mentioned, once I got a medical diagnosis, I noticed myself being a little less critical and a bit more compassionate toward my body. I mean, it was fighting a disease, for heaven's sake. And I felt challenged to consider this question: *What would happen if I spent more time caring for my body than criticizing it?*

So I decided to find out. Instead of wasting a bunch of energy being mad at, criticizing, or comparing my body, I started investing that energy into caring for it. This is around the time I began to learn how to support my hormones and feminine physiology. I actually listened to my body when it was needing rest or lighter movement than high-intensity cardio or fitness training. I started my days with the sun instead of a screen. I created a simple non-toxic bedtime skin-care routine as a way to unwind and because it made me happy.

I was also challenged to be more thoughtful about how I was speaking about my body. In a conversation with a counselor I was meeting with at the time, she suggested that even a small tweak in how I talked about the health-related challenges I was facing could make a big difference in how I was feeling mentally, emotionally, and perhaps even physically (which makes sense, given that those elements really are so intricately connected).

It's not your body's fault. It's sin's fault—it's the result of the Fall. And your body isn't broken. It was designed with the brilliance and glory of heaven. But it *does* live in a fallen world, and that means it will be touched by brokenness.

"Instead of saying 'my acne' or 'my endometriosis' or whatever the issue you're facing is, try just saying 'my skin is struggling with acne' or 'the endometriosis I was diagnosed with.'" Then she continued, "How we speak about an issue we are facing reflects our beliefs about that issue. And sometimes, without even realizing it, we begin to identify with that issue. We make acne *our* acne, as if it's a part of who we are. But it's not. It's a symptom or struggle we may currently have, but it is not part of who we are. How we think and speak can slowly shape our beliefs, and we have to be mindful of these things."

That's so true! I thought. *And I've been believing my body is the problem and I've been acting like the challenges I'm facing are part of me—as if they're my identity. The truth is, they are simply a challenge, or a circumstance, that I'm facing.*

Even the Bible speaks to the truth of that: "Death and life are in the power of the tongue, and those who love it will eat its fruits" (Proverbs 18:21). There is power in our words. And although we may not think much about words when it comes to caring for our bodies, the thoughts we have and words we speak are truly at the foundation of it all. Why? Because what we believe will directly influence what we do and how we treat our bodies.

If we believe and speak life and truth, that will elicit a response of caring for our bodies as part of God's good creation. If we believe and speak death and lies, that will elicit a response of criticism and even a hyperfixation on whatever it is we're criticizing.

The world will tell you everything that's wrong with your body and sell you on how it can be fixed with a pill, potion, product, or procedure.

But the truth is, your body needs to be supported, not fixed.

And although there are absolutely times that quality products like natural skin care and some procedures (such as to repair an ailment or diagnose or repair disease such as endometriosis) can be helpful or even necessary, the best way to support your body is to speak truth, be gentle and patient with it, and regularly give it the good things God made.

BEING GOOD TO YOUR BODY MEANS BELIEVING THE TRUTH ABOUT YOUR IDENTITY

As I thought about what my counselor said regarding how we speak about ourselves, I realized how much my beliefs can shape whether caring for my body and well-being leads to freedom or bondage.

When we begin to believe the lie that the flaws, symptoms, and diagnoses we're facing are part of who we are—if we make them our identity—then in our efforts to address or fix it, we can quickly head toward idolatry. The pursuit of health and healing can become an obsession or, as Tim Keller calls idols, a "counterfeit god."[2]

Where we place our identity reveals what we worship, and what we worship reveals where we place our trust. If my identity is firmly rooted in the One who made me, there also will be my worship (and my trust). If my identity is rooted in my body, there also will be my worship (and my trust will be in myself).

When I was struggling with recurrent miscarriages, I began to feel like "the miscarriage girl." There was a time that whenever I thought about myself and my body, the first thing that came to mind was the lie that "I'm the girl who can't carry a baby to save her life." That false identity was steering me toward making an idol out of my body and my pursuit of healing.

Checking ourselves and coming back to the truth of who God says we are, not what our pain or circumstances make us believe, is critical if we truly want to be good to our bodies.

WHO DOES GOD SAY WE ARE?

We can go back to the very first chapter of God's Word and see that we were made in His image (see Genesis 1:27). Scripture also calls us God's children (see John 1:12), chosen (see 1 Peter 2:9), and citizens of heaven (see Philippians 3:20).

The health challenges you may be facing—whether chronic illness, infertility, or something else—are not your identity, not part of who you are. And being gluten-free or vegan or whatever other lifestyle choice you make is not your identity. It cannot be. The moment being "crunchy" is elevated above being created by the God of the universe, or holistic living is elevated over being who you are in Christ, things get messy. Worship gets misplaced.

Look, you are a daughter of the King. And when you believe that truth in your heart, you will be able to treat your body accordingly—not like an idol, but like royalty, as described in 1 Peter 2:9: If you are in Christ, "you are a chosen people, a royal priesthood, a holy nation, God's special possession, that you may declare the praises of him" (NIV).

> Care for your body well—to bring Him glory, not to fix everything about yourself. Your heart—your body— is a temple of the Holy Spirit, the place where God Himself chooses to dwell.

And that means that as a daughter of the King, perfect health and total restoration are the inheritance that awaits you on the other side of heaven, for eternity. Your ultimate hope is not in health, healing, or achieving the ideal body in this life.

So while you're here on earth, care for your body well—to bring Him glory, not to fix everything about yourself. Your heart—your body—is a temple of the Holy Spirit, the place where God Himself chooses to dwell.

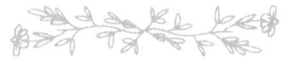

PRAYER

Father, I confess that I have believed lies about my body and put my identity in the wrong things. I humbly ask for Your grace and guidance to help me keep my heart and mind aligned with the truth of who You say I am. Please help me run everything I begin to believe about my body through the lens of Scripture instead of the lens of societal norms or my feelings. Amen.

PRACTICAL APPLICATION

Reflect on lies you may be believing about your body. What is the feature you criticize or symptom you complain about the most? Is it your nose? Weight? Do you have chronic pain or struggle with acne? How can you shift the way you speak about that thing so your words and attitude speak life over your body? What is one thing you can do to care for your body whenever you are about to criticize or complain about it? For example, whenever you criticize your skin for having acne, pause and redirect the time you spend criticizing into caring for your skin, such as by hydrating, eating a nourishing meal, or doing your skin-care routine.

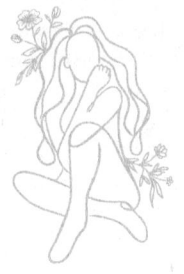

Chapter 6

SHED THE SHAME

I didn't know it was possible to experience mom guilt before actually experiencing motherhood, but I did. It sounds kind of weird when I say it out loud, but allow me to explain what I mean.

When I went through recurrent miscarriages, I couldn't help but feel a sense of guilt or shame each time I lost a baby. As much as I logically knew that it wasn't my fault, it was hard not to believe there was something wrong with me. I wondered if maybe I was being punished. I felt as though my body, which *should* be the safest place for my children to be, was not a safe place for them to grow and thrive.

And in many ways, it was embarrassing. When people asked if I had any kids or if we planned to have kids, I felt ashamed to admit what I was experiencing. And I think perhaps part of why I felt that way was because our fertility challenge was technically on *my* side. Everything was perfectly healthy on the male side of the equation. We would conceive, and then everything would go haywire within my body.

So while my husband never put any blame whatsoever on me, I deeply wrestled with the lie that I was failing to give him babies. Something within me and inside my body was failing my family.

That was an extremely heavy burden to carry. On top of that, my face and sometimes my shoulders were chronically broken out with acne. I felt gross and, quite frankly, ugly—the furthest thing from feminine or womanly.

Like I said, logically I knew those were all lies straight from the pit of hell and mouth of the Enemy. If a friend of mine were struggling with those thoughts, I would have been able to speak so much truth into her heart. But when I felt those things myself, logic went out the window and it was such a different story. The lies felt so true sometimes and were hard to shake.

At first, I thought that I felt *guilt*—mom guilt for my body seemingly failing, and guilt for not being able to give my husband children—but I later realized that I was actually experiencing *shame*.

Guilt and shame can seem similar but are not the same. Guilt is a focus on behavior, whereas shame is a focus on the self, or identity. Brené Brown explains it like this: "Shame is 'I am bad'; guilt is 'I did something bad.'"[1]

Psychologist Robert Karen identified four categories of shame: existential, situational, class, and narcissistic.[2] In my case, I felt existential shame, which occurs when we become self-aware of an objective, unpleasant truth about ourselves or our situation.

I was facing an unpleasant truth about myself and my situation: I was covered in cystic acne, and babies were not surviving in my body. That quickly spiraled into the belief that mine must be a bad body.

This shame was part of the driving force behind my desire for solutions, which turned into a pretty intense pursuit of healing. Of course, my desire for a family and the instinct to protect any future babies I might conceive were also part of my motivation.

Although the desire to heal and protect my family was good and honorable, shame was still in there. It was part of it, whether I wanted to admit it or not. And I think if people were honest with themselves, many would find what sometimes drives their health journey or the ways they try to change, fix, or heal their bodies is shame.

For example, many people strive to lose weight and get in great shape, most likely so they feel better, have energy and strength to keep up with their kids, or to care for their cardiovascular health. But sometimes there's another driving factor that keeps them from ordering dessert and helps them get up for those early-morning gym sessions: shame. Perhaps words spoken to them throughout their lives about their weight or appearance—whether by others, themselves, or both—is part of that shame.

Why do you think the message to "prove the haters wrong" that seems to circulate through all the personal-development, fitness, and motivational subculture is so popular? It speaks to something deep inside us, where the voices that hurt us, made us feel less than, or caused us to question our worth once spoke. So the phrase works. It's a powerful motivator because it touches a place in our hearts where we have felt shame, where we have received and possibly even believed lies, or where we've identified with what has been spoken over us by others (or perhaps even by ourselves).

Logically, if the words and the lies that have been spewed at us held no weight, why would we need to prove anything to those people? Why would we feel motivated to prove them wrong?

We wouldn't.

So, I would argue that messaging like that motivates because it speaks to our insecurity—the places deep inside us where we've felt shame and allowed the lies spoken to us ("You're not pretty," "You're fat," "Your arms look weird") to shape our identity.

Maybe weight loss or fitness isn't part of your journey. It may not be an area in which you've believed lies or experienced shame. Perhaps it's something else. Maybe you've dealt with acne, infertility, a disability, or another physical challenge that you feel makes your body weak, unattractive, or broken.

Shame says, "You are broken, ugly, and unlovable. Your body isn't good and needs to be fixed." Scripture says, "You are chosen and loved. Your body, though not perfect, is a God-given gift."

And as great as it can be to pay attention to symptoms your body presents, address root causes, and work toward restoration or healing, I know from personal experience that when those issues are rooted in shame, it's easy for a good intention to become an obsession.

Shame says, "You are broken, ugly, and unlovable. Your body is bad and needs to be fixed." Scripture says, "You are chosen and loved. Your body, though not perfect, is a God-given gift."

Sometimes the line between shame and Scripture can be hard to see. Often, they spark similar actions, such as eating better, getting into a workout routine, and creating a healthier environment. But here's the difference: When our healthy habits and journey to wellness are driven by shame, we are so much more likely to get caught in the shame cycle. Nothing will ever be enough. We measure our worth by the outcomes we can achieve: how much weight was lost, how well the hormones balanced, whether or not we could clear our skin or get pregnant or do whatever other desired thing we want to achieve.

But when the way we care for our bodies is founded on the truth of Scripture, we can make changes and efforts through the lens of stewardship, which brings freedom and balance instead of obsession or striving toward perfection. We can make healthy swaps and implement disciplines that benefit our physical well-being without putting our entire hope in those things or whether we achieve the outcome—the clear skin, the pregnancy, the slimmer waist—we'd like to achieve.

> Being as healthy as possible is critical to fulfilling our callings well, but being healthy is not the calling itself.

Instead of health or a health outcome being the end or goal itself (which really just turns it into an obsession), healthy living should be a means to an end. Being as healthy as possible is critical to fulfilling our callings well, but being healthy is not the calling itself.

Ultimately, the heart posture by which we pursue health deeply influences whether being good to our bodies becomes an obsession or an act of obedience and whether it serves God or serves ourselves. Scripture says to treat our bodies like temples, not idols, and it's only possible to do that when none but God is on the throne of our hearts.

WHEN YOU DON'T SEE RESULTS RIGHT AWAY

Have you ever set out on a health-related journey with a goal in mind—losing weight, clearing your skin, healing chronic pain, or something else—only to feel as though you keep coming up short?

I have.

Sometimes being good to my body, figuring out what on earth it's trying to tell me and how I can give it what it needs, seems harder than trying to decipher the Da Vinci code.

When I was trying to get to the bottom of my acne situation and fertility struggles, it felt like a whole lot of trial and error, starts and restarts. Just when I thought I was making progress, I'd have a setback or get stuck. It was exhausting and a little embarrassing. *Why can't I figure this out?* I'd wonder. *What am I missing?*

While shame can often be a sneaky motivator behind our pursuit of health, fitness, or healing, it can also come up if we don't see the results we hope for very quickly.

Why? Because even if we are being as intentional as possible, when our best efforts seem to amount to nothing, we begin to believe *we* are the problem. When we do all the right things and don't see the results we hope for, it's easy to believe there must be something wrong with us or that we are failing.

Now, is it possible that lack of discipline or consistency can be the reason for the lack of change we'd like to see? Or maybe just having the wrong information and therefore doing the wrong things? Of course. Many times that is the case.

But what about when we are being as diligent and consistent as possible and our efforts just don't seem to yield much fruit? What about when we nourish our bodies with real food, move regularly, spend months or years undergoing what feels like endless testing, and do all the "right" things, only to still not get pregnant or experience the hoped-for healing and feel like it's all for nothing? When we're disciplined and consistent but get thrown off course by a surprise circumstance, our family's needs, or even a tragedy?

It's discouraging. I felt that way when I first began to make healthy lifestyle changes and yet we still lost one more baby. And then my acne, which had improved for a bit, came back in full force shortly after that loss. Words can hardly describe the sheer defeat I felt, like all my efforts had been in vain.

And those situations? The ones where we do our best and it just doesn't seem to make an ounce of difference? They plant the lie that we are failing—that *we're the problem.* That's what shame does.

It's sneaky, and just as much as it can be a motivator, it can also be a demotivator. And as time goes on, we may be tempted to think that we might as well give up—that because we can't visibly see any significant impact from our efforts, we must be wasting our time.

But we're human. We're complex beings. There's a lot that even science and medicine don't understand about our bodies. Only God knows. As much as we'd love for it to be as simple as $A + B = C$, sometimes the journey feels more like $A + B = LMNOPQRSTUV$.

That is why we can't afford to not lean on His sovereignty. We cannot rely on self-sufficiency—it will get us only so far.

When we give our best efforts and our body just does not seem to be cooperating, that is *not* the time to give up or neglect it, although it can be tempting to do just that. Every single positive step we take to support our bodies counts. Whether or not the pounds fall off or the problem we're dealing with gets resolved in the way or by the time we think it should, it is not our job to fix everything or achieve the perfect or ideal body. It is our job to be good to our imperfect bodies; give them good, God-made things; and depend on God's wisdom and sovereignty on every step of the journey.

> It is not our job to fix everything or achieve the perfect or ideal body. It is our job to be good to our imperfect bodies; give them good, God-made things; and depend on God's wisdom and sovereignty on every step of the journey.

Maybe God isn't asking you to do it all perfectly or achieve a desired outcome, however good that outcome may be. Maybe, just maybe, He's asking you to care for the vessel He's given you to the best of your ability and trust Him on the journey, regardless of the outcome.

See the difference? It's subtle. It's easy to miss. But it makes an incredible difference in whether our pursuit of health and well-being is done from a place of surrender and stewardship—"Everything I have is Yours, God, and I trust You"—or from a place of striving and self-sufficiency—*It's all up to me; I have to fix it myself.*

Discipline with a healthy dependency on God leads to freedom and can help us continue to be good to our bodies despite the outcome. Shame, on the other hand, leads to striving and self-sufficiency. When we don't get the results we expect to see, it can be utterly defeating and can dare us to completely give up on being good to our bodies.

THE BIBLE AND BODY SHAME

I find it so interesting to go back to the Garden of Eden and examine humanity's very first experience with shame. Before sin entered the picture, Adam and Eve were not aware of their nakedness. They did not feel the need to cover their bodies, nor did they even think about it. There was nothing corrupted about the body, and they were free to live and be, never overanalyzing or feeling shame about their bodies.

Enter sin.

Immediately after they sinned against God, Adam and Eve became aware of their bodies and their nakedness, or their vulnerability. Their entire being went from flawless (without sin or shame) to fallen (touched by sin and, therefore, shame).

I'd argue they felt both guilt and shame: guilt because of the awareness that they had *done* something wrong (behavior), which then led to shame (the sense that they *are* something wrong, no longer perfectly united with their creator but now fallen sinners). And as a result, they had a sudden need to cover themselves and hide—a need that did not exist before.

We can't escape the fact that the sin that now touches all of humanity, and the shame that accompanies it, led to a direct awareness and response to hide when it came to the body.

Adam and Eve were aware of and ashamed of their nakedness only *after* the Fall, as sin made them aware of their vulnerability and shortcomings, something that before was not even a thought. Brokenness within our bodies—health issues such as pain, diseases, or infertility—feel like vulnerabilities. They are areas in which we feel exposed and possibly even weak. Similarly, because of the Fall, we have an acute awareness of our nakedness, or the things we don't like about ourselves.

In an article with a biblical take on body shame, Jaquelle Crowe explains that "God created our physical bodies and declared them good (Genesis 1:31). But in the frustration of shame, we're tempted to hate our bodies (Genesis 3:7). They become the problem and the enemy." Crowe continues, "We act like teenage Gnostics, believing the body is arbitrarily evil and we need to be released from it. But the problem is not with our bodies; it's with our perspective—a perspective shot through with sin. We loathe our bodies because we've mistaken God's gift as a curse."[3]

Woof. The truth is, chronic illness, infertility, or the shape of our nose isn't really the problem, although it may seem like it is. It's evidence of the real problem, which is sin. And body shame, when we dislike or hate our bodies, makes our bodies the focus.

Even if we don't like something about our bodies, the fixation on them—and perhaps even on fixing or changing them—can quickly turn them into idols, the objects of our worship. And that is the exact opposite purpose of the bodies we are given.

First Corinthians 6:20 says to glorify God in our bodies, which tells me that the purpose of the body is to worship, not to be worshipped. The purpose of the body is not to look a certain way but rather to *live* a certain way—to fulfill our God-given callings. The whole point of caring for our health is not to maintain an image but to mirror the image of God.

I love what my friend Jess Connolly says in an article talking about her book *Breaking Free from Body Shame:*

> The truest thing about you is that you are made and loved by God. And the truest thing about Him is that He cannot make bad things.
>
> Far from a superficial issue, self-image is a *spiritual* issue, because God has named your body good from the beginning.[4]

Shewwwww. Pin that on my forehead, please and thank you.

Did you catch that last part? Don't skim over it. We could find a dozen places in Scripture that tell us the truth about our bodies, but if we look solely at the Creation account, God called everything He created "good." The human body was part of that creation. You and I—our good bodies—are a part of that creation, friend.

> The purpose of the body is not to look a certain way but rather to *live* a certain way—to fulfill our God-given callings.

Have they since been touched by sin? Yes.

Are they perfect? No.

Will they be free of blemish or brokenness? Unfortunately, no. But that's not because they are the problem or bad. It's because sin is the problem and brings bad things, such as flaws, sickness, and death.

Your body lives in a world that is fallen, which means it will be touched by brokenness. But that doesn't make it a bad body.

BEING GOOD TO YOUR BODY
IS SHEDDING SHAME

I was eleven years old when a neighbor girl told me I had thunder thighs. And I believed her. Looking back at photos of my eleven-year-old self, the last thing I see is thunder thighs. I mean, I had an athletic body type, but my legs were the furthest thing from being large.

Yet her words cut deep, and I believed them as gospel truth for a good portion of my adolescent and young adult life.

I've come a long way since then, but even in my thirties, I still sometimes find myself overthinking how my legs appear. It's wild how difficult it can be to shake the lies spoken over us early in life.

If all that God created (including our bodies) is called good by the Creator Himself, then being good to our bodies, even when we don't like a feature or we try to heal something that seems to be malfunctioning, requires that we consistently revisit truth.

The first question we have to ask ourselves is, *Do I take God at His word?*

In other words, *Do I believe that all that He created, including my body, is good?*

If I agree with the creator of every good and perfect thing that my body is part of His good creation, that means it is worthy of being given the good things He created for its thriving.

And it's my job to shed the shame so I can give the good body God gave me the good things He made. Not because I did anything to deserve them, but because He did everything to freely give them.

The second question we have to ask ourselves when it comes to how we view and therefore care for our bodies is, *Am I doing this [diet, fitness plan, protocol] to glorify my body for the sake of what it can do for me or to glorify the God who gave me this body for the sake of fulfilling His calling for me?*

My body is a gift and a blessing. But unlike everything the world says, being good to our bodies requires that we view them appropriately. It means agreeing with our creator that although humanity and sin may corrupt it, all that God created is good, including our bodies. And then it's not being preoccupied by them—caring for them, yes, but not beating them into submission or obsessing over every imperfection. The more we fixate on our bodies—whether on the things we love, the things we hate, the things we want to make different, or the things that make us feel shame—the less capacity we have to partake in the change we were born to help make in this world.

When we view our bodies rightly, ultimately as His and as good, God-given gifts, we can care for them accordingly. Not to achieve perfect health or the ideal image, but instead to fulfill our callings.

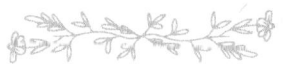

PRAYER

God, please reveal where shame may be fueling how I am treating my body. I want to have the eyes to see where certain habits and disciplines (or lack thereof) are driven by shame instead of truth. I know that my body is far from perfect and will be touched by brokenness on this side of heaven, but I believe that everything You created—including my body—is good and is worthy of good things. Give me peace and clarity and help me live aligned with that belief so I can care for my body the right way. Amen.

PRACTICAL APPLICATION

Examine your motives. What is driving your health journey (or lack thereof)? Is shame pushing you to strive for certain outcomes or perhaps neglect your body altogether? Consider inviting two or three trusted people—close friends, a mentor, your spouse—to honestly speak into that and tell you what they see driving the choices (good or bad) you make for your body.

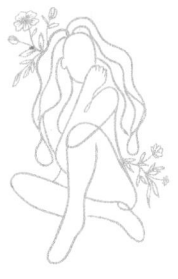

Chapter 7

KEEP IT SIMPLE

I cut out dairy because I heard it was inflammatory. Then, as I was sipping an almond-milk smoothie while scrolling online, I came across a post that linked to an article about why almond milk may not actually be healthy.

You've got to be kidding me.

This wasn't the first time something like that happened either. A few months prior, I had reduced my intake of carbs because, well, keto, right? Not long after that, I found another school of thought that explains why we actually need a decent amount of carbs because our cells run on glucose. And then everyone and their mother on social media started making sourdough and talking about all the benefits of fermented bread.

I started taking prenatal vitamins, but of course I came across information all about why I should maybe reconsider doing that too. I bought an air purifier, only to then come across a thousand other gadgets I supposedly needed, from acupressure mats to frequency patches and a thousand other tools to try. I could give more examples, but you probably get the point. Every time I thought I'd made a healthy change, I'd stumble upon a study or post that let me know the change may not actually be very healthy.

Raise your hand if you've ever experienced something like that. Go on, raise it. I can't be alone in this! It's frustrating to feel like no matter what you do, there's always more you could do or that there's always someone doing more. There's always another perspective, making you rethink everything. It can be so overwhelming, right?

Frustrated, I tossed my phone onto the couch. I mean, is almond milk healthy or not?!

TIMELESS VERSUS TRENDS

Honestly, I don't know that I have the answer to the almond-milk question. I have my thoughts on it but I'm not sure that even really matters. What does matter is that we keep things simple. We live in the information age, which means we are susceptible to information overload, and that can very quickly distract us from the timeless disciplines that are most beneficial to our health. While we may all have our preferences or ideas regarding certain things, identifying them can help separate the timeless from the trendy— the basics from the extras. That is important because it can be so tempting to jump to something that may absolutely be healthy but not totally necessary and perhaps even kind of faddish. For example, buying a fancy red-light machine might be beneficial; I'm personally a huge advocate for red light therapy. *But* if you're not even opening your windows or getting outside daily or setting boundaries on screen time before bed, you're skipping right over the most basic, timeless (and free) things you could be doing to support your body.

In a world of endless fads and health trends, my best advice to reduce overwhelm is to prioritize the big stuff first—the biblical habits that keep your body living aligned with your God-given design. So let's revisit the basics.

WHAT'S TIMELESS?

If you were about to embark on a health journey and ask me right now, "Where should I start?" I'd tell you to start with the basics.

That may feel a bit repetitive since we discussed the biblical principles for well-being in chapter 3, but this is on purpose. I want to continue to reiterate these basic, biblical, timeless things to help us avoid getting too caught up in information overload or every new trend that might be helpful but not totally necessary.

What are some of the most basic basics?

- **Hydrate.** Filter some of the junk out of your water, as most of our exposure to toxins comes from what we eat and drink. Nowadays, most tap water is riddled with toxins that it would be best not to consume multiple times per day. Check out ClearlyFiltered.com for water filtration systems and filtered water bottles. Throw in a pinch of sea salt for extra hydration.
- **Replenish minerals and eat real food.** Less takeout and packaged food processed with chemicals, more home-cooked meals with simple ingredients and foods in their whole form.
- **Support your sleep and circadian rhythms.** Less blue light and more sunlight. Try an earlier bedtime. Shut off Netflix and prioritize quality sleep. (If you have a baby,

you get a bit of a pass here!) Bottom line: Create regular rhythms of rest.

- **Spend time in nature.** Get outside, breathe fresh air, take deep breaths, spend time in sunlight, and walk barefoot.
- **Move your body.** You don't need a fancy gym membership or workout equipment. Go for walks, stretch, jog, swim, play with your kids, dance—do whatever works for you. Just move. Every single day, somehow, someway.
- **Be in community with God and people.** Read your Bible, listen to worship music, share a meal with friends, know your neighbors, and get plugged into your local community. Your physical health is directly connected to your spiritual, emotional, mental, and relational health. Remember Genesis 2:18? We are made for community.
- **Cultivate a life-giving environment.** Reduce toxins where you can, let the natural light in, tidy up before bed each night, and maybe get some plants or fresh-cut flowers. If you want to be fruitful and feel full of life, make sure the environment around you is fruitful and life-giving to support that. Just like God instructed the very first humans to tend to the place around them, the garden, we must tend to and cultivate the environment we're placed in (see Genesis 2:15).

WHAT'S EXTRA?

Basically everything else is extra. Okay, maybe that's a little dramatic, but here's a short list of examples of health-related trends that can be beneficial for some (but harmful for others) and probably aren't absolute necessities for most (at least not for extended periods of time):

- fad diets—Paleo, keto, Whole30, and so on
- intermittent fasting
- countless supplements
- wearable wellness tech (such as an Apple Watch)
- cold plunges
- saunas
- counting every macro
- glucose/blood sugar monitoring (unless directed by a doctor)
- fancy gym memberships

The list could go on, but you probably get the idea.

Does that mean we shouldn't use any of these tools or things? Of course not! Like I said, they absolutely *can* be beneficial. But I'd still put them in the "extra" category because I'd rather you just start doing the most fundamental things without stressing yourself out trying to keep up with every new study or buying all the latest tools and expensive gadgets.

BEING GOOD TO YOUR BODY BEGINS WITH THE BASICS

The bottom line is that being good to your body is truly one small step at a time, and the first steps should always be the basics—the biblical foundations. And if you're stressed-out trying to do all the things, go *back* to the basics.

> You cannot be holistically well if your pursuit of physical health is harming your spiritual, mental, or relational health.

Perhaps the hardest lesson I learned on my journey is this: You cannot be holistically well if your pursuit of physical health is harming your spiritual, mental, or relational health. It's all integrally connected. And the amount we can do for our physical health may vary season to season. There may be seasons in which we have more time and resources to invest in some of the trendier or "extra" things, and when we can, that's great! Those things will absolutely bless our bodies, as long as doing them doesn't totally stress us out.

There will likely be other times when all we can manage to maintain is the basics. And that's totally okay too. If we can manage to keep the basics as our baseline, we're going to be all right.

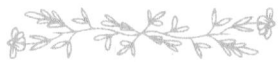

PRAYER

Lord, I admit that sometimes I fail to be disciplined and give my body the basic good things You made. Help me be a better steward right where I am. From this point on, I commit to prioritizing the simple things before I get too tangled up in or carried away with all the fads and extras the world has to offer. Please help me see where I need to take ownership of my well-being and improve how I'm doing the most basic things my body needs. Amen.

PRACTICAL APPLICATION

Look through this checklist of the basics. Before you get too caught up in doing or buying all the extras, ask yourself if you're regularly doing these foundational things—if you're giving your body *these* things. Go ahead—run through the list. If there are any boxes you don't check off, make it your goal to focus on establishing *those* habits over the next few weeks.

☐ *I meet my body's hydration needs, ideally with filtered and re-mineralized water.*

☐ *I cook at least 70 to 80 percent of my meals at home with real, whole food ingredients.*

☐ *I eat three balanced meals per day with nourishing snacks between (no skipping meals).*

☐ *I have a consistent bedtime routine and get at least seven hours of sleep each night.*

☐ *I turn off blue light and screens at least thirty to sixty minutes before bed each night.*

☐ *I get sunlight in my eyes first thing in the morning (step outside or open a window, no devices for at least thirty minutes after waking).*

☐ *I spend time outside and get fresh air daily.*

☐ *I am active and intentionally move my body daily (physically active job, formal workout, or simply a walk after supper).*

☐ *I connect with my local community weekly.*

☐ *I prioritize daily prayer and time with God.*

☐ *I ensure that my home is as healthy of an environment as possible (let natural light in, reduce toxins where and when possible, crack a window or use an air purifier to filter the air).*

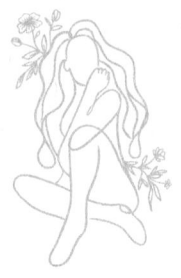

Chapter 8

REDUCE YOUR BURDEN

As I've mentioned already, chronic cystic acne has been a big part of my health journey. I tried what felt like every acne skin-care product I could find, but it seemed like my skin just got worse. It was frustrating and embarrassing, and I had no idea what was going on with me, especially before I did further testing and got an endometriosis diagnosis.

I cycled through skin treatments and dermatologist visits, but I didn't even consider that the acne might be connected to something internally—until I experienced miscarriages and infertility. That is when I really started to look deeper and consider root issues. It dawned on me that maybe some of the symptoms I was having were smoke signals my body was trying to send me.

Up until that point in my journey, I had been more reactive than proactive. I was treating rather than preventing. If a pimple appeared, I'd pop and treat it with a spot treatment. But for several years, I never took the time to investigate root causes or do the work to address what may have been going on within my body.

It wasn't until whatever was "off" in my body started to break my heart and affect my starting a family that I began to take it more seriously. Isn't that sad? Instead of listening to the signs my body was sending me, it wasn't until I went through something traumatic that I began to take my health more seriously.

Unfortunately, that is an all-too-common experience. Most people I know who have made significant changes to their lifestyles to support their bodies from the inside out have done so after a very painful, jarring experience, whether it was a chronic illness, miscarriage, or scary diagnosis.

If we're not in any kind of significant pain or facing anything debilitating or devastating, it's far too easy to assume we are "fine" and put our well-being on the back burner, until our bodies practically have to scream at us to get our attention.

As I ruthlessly investigated what was going on with my body, perhaps one of the most upsetting things I uncovered was the truth about the majority of products being sold on shelves (and that I owned and used every day!).

I learned that most conventional personal-care and household products are made with countless harmful ingredients—such as parabens and phthalates—with no disclaimer or warning to consumers. Many of those ingredients have endocrine-disrupting properties and are known allergens and even known carcinogens.

I was genuinely shocked.

Wait, so these big corporations don't actually care about the safety of their products or health of their customers? I wondered as I walked through the beauty aisles of the local convenience stores. _Is it really all about achieving mass production and maximizing profit?_

I wasn't sure I was convinced, because I didn't want to believe it, so I did more research.

I learned about various chemicals of concern and common

products they're often found in. For example, "1,4-dioxane is a contaminant linked to cancer found in products that create suds, such as shampoo and liquid soap."[1] And parabens, a class of preservatives found in a wide array of cosmetic and personal-care products, not only "are potential endocrine disruptors due to their ability to mimic estrogen" but also have been linked to developmental and reproductive toxicity.[2] Those are just a couple of examples from a long list of studies I dived into.

Then my next thought became, *Well, the amounts of these ingredients are probably not very big. Most of these products are just using small amounts of parabens or other concerning ingredients. It certainly can't be enough to be harmful, right?*

The Campaign for Safe Cosmetics (CSC) puts the answer to that question this way: "Because the body's own hormones convey messages throughout the body in tiny amounts, extremely low levels of toxic chemicals, including many of those used in personal care products, may have serious effects on metabolism, reproductive development, and risks for later life disease."[3]

Welp, there's that. Plus, I had to consider if it were really as small of an exposure as I thought it was.

I mean, sure, if I were using only a couple of products with small amounts of these concerning ingredients, that would be one thing. But if many of these ingredients were in practically all the products I was using every single day, that isn't so insignificant. It's repeated exposure daily, from many different products I'm using on my body and in my home. And that adds up!

I was so disappointed. I had been buying and trusting countless products with ingredients like those for years, and I felt lied to—deceived, really. Like most women, I had been led to believe that if it was sold on a shelf, it must be safe.

And once my eyes were opened to all this information, I couldn't unknow it. I couldn't unsee it. So I promptly threw out half my products and began to overhaul practically every semi-toxic thing I owned (which seemed like everything).

OBEDIENCE OVER OBSESSION

Between swapping most of my personal-care and household products, learning to read labels, and making safer purchases, I made a lot of progress toward reducing my body's toxin burden. And in many ways, that was incredibly beneficial for my hormonal health and overall well-being.

Admittedly, though, the more I learned about all the places toxins can be hiding (in the most basic things, such as water and air and even our favorite undies), it seemed like what started as good and worthy intentions began to spiral into fear and obsession.

It wasn't even that choosing safer swaps or investing in a water filter was wrong or bad. On the contrary, those are very good things to do. It was that my heart and mind had begun to shift into an unhealthy place. I felt constantly stressed and crippled with fear, and I took it upon myself to avoid every last toxin.

For a time, I managed to sustain this way of living. I stopped getting my nails done because of the fumes, even though a manicure was something I enjoyed now and then. I diligently researched every item I considered buying to make sure it was as clean as could be.

Although sometimes a short season of tenacity, diligence, and discipline like that can be necessary for healing, I don't believe being that strict is sustainable for a long period of time or as a lifestyle. Here's why: At some point along the way, I looked up from my pursuit of avoiding all the "bad" stuff and realized I wasn't having very much fun. I wasn't really living fully in the freedom

Christ offered me. The Bible says in 2 Corinthians 3:17, "Where the Spirit of the Lord is, there is freedom." And Galatians 5:1 tells us, "For freedom Christ has set us free; stand firm therefore, and do not submit again to a yoke of slavery." But I wasn't living as someone who had been set free; I was living in bondage.

Now, for context, the slavery we are set free from according to the Bible is the slavery of sin. And making anything, even a good thing like low-tox living, an idol that takes the place of God on the throne of your heart *is* sin.

Although I had good intentions and made these changes for good reasons, I couldn't deny that I was at risk of slipping into idolatry. As much as I was trying to be a good steward of my body, I had crossed over into allowing fear to drive me into obsession instead of allowing the freedom I had in Christ to lead me toward obedience.

Caring for our bodies, which the Bible calls temples of the Holy Spirit, is an act of obedience.

Obedience? Yes, obedience. Caring for our bodies, which the Bible calls temples of the Holy Spirit, is an act of obedience. In 1 Corinthians 10:31, Paul tells us, "Whether you eat or drink, or whatever you do, do all to the glory of God." Everything we do—including how we treat our bodies and what we use and consume—should be done for the glory of God.

So yes, being thoughtful about caring for our bodies is an act of obedience. But if we're not careful or have zero accountability, our sinful tendency toward idolatry can distort a good thing and make it into a god thing.

Unintentionally, the ruthless pursuit of reducing toxins was becoming a god to me. But intentional or not, when health or healing takes God's rightful place on the throne of our hearts—when it's where we place our hope—it is no longer healthy. That doesn't make it unimportant; it simply means we need to recalibrate our heart posture and motives.

STRESS IS A TOXIN TOO

I have a question. If we are doing something to support our physical well-being, such as reducing our toxin burden, but it becomes so stressful that it harms our mental and spiritual well-being, is it still good for our bodies?

I'd argue that at least some of the benefit that may come from reducing toxic chemicals is lost when it's done from a place of stress, anxiety, or obsession. Why? Because although the body may have fewer chemical toxins, it is now going to have to deal with elevated cortisol from being perpetually in fight-or-flight mode.

That's not just my opinion. Research has shown numerous effects of stress on the body's well-being. Stress that gets out of hand can lead to everything from digestive and sleep problems to high blood pressure, fatigue, and diabetes.[4] In fact, stress can even negatively affect our menstrual cycles and reproductive health. According to the American Psychological Association (APA),

> High levels of stress may be associated with absent or irregular menstrual cycles, more painful periods, and changes in the length of cycles. . . .
>
> Stress can negatively impact a woman's ability to conceive, the health of her pregnancy, and her postpartum adjustment.[5]

The absolute irony in my case was that I was stressing myself out trying to avoid all toxins that could hurt my fertility and, in the process, creating stress in my body—which can also have a negative impact on reproductive health and pregnancy. What a catch-22.

I mean, what's a gal to do? Can we even win here? How do we reduce the amount of endocrine disruptors, carcinogens, and other harmful substances that we're exposed to on a daily basis without becoming so stressed-out that we end up creating another problem altogether?

Here's what I'll say: I don't think the answer is to throw in the towel and not take any steps toward reducing toxin exposure just because it's possible that it *might* become stressful. Although stress poses a burden to our bodies, so do toxic chemicals. And toxins are everywhere, so it *is* wise to reduce what we can, where we can.

Here's a visual that can be helpful to come back to when struggling to find that balance: Think of your body as a bathtub that is filling with water. The water represents toxins: hormone disruptors, carcinogens, and more. The tub has a drain, which represents your body's natural detox functions (like your liver is responsible for). The body is made to detox just like the bathtub is made to drain. If the bathtub is filling at a manageable rate and the drain is open, the drain will be able to do its job and the tub won't overflow. But if there is far too much water filling the tub faster than the drain can remove it, the tub water will overflow.

That is kind of what happens when we're overloaded with toxin exposure, which, in our modern world and environment, most of us are. Our bodies are designed to be able to detox to a certain degree, which means we don't have to avoid every possible exposure. And that's good news because total avoidance wouldn't be possible anyway. But if our detox pathways are not supported or are overloaded with toxins through our food, environments, water, and everyday products, issues can arise much faster.

So the goal is not necessarily to completely empty the tub but rather to reduce the toxin load, or slow down that flow of water, so our bodies can keep up and detox the exposures we cannot avoid. What we're aiming for is not total avoidance of toxins, just reduction of them. And where we can't reduce or swap something, our next best option is to support our detox pathways, such as by sweating and moving our bodies, staying hydrated, doing lymphatic massages, or eating fiber-rich whole foods.

That said, I would love to tell you there's a simple solution, such as to swap some magic number of products (and not one more or one less), and you'll find that perfect balance. But the fact is, it is so individual, as we all have different capacities and thresholds due to many variables, such as season of life and existing obligations, budget and ability to access and afford certain products, and the support system an individual has or doesn't have (for example, a spouse who is on board or not). What is stressful to one person may not be as stressful to another. Making five to ten swaps to safer products might feel very easy and manageable to someone who has a flexible budget and a supportive spouse, whereas making just a few swaps may feel overwhelming to someone who already has several other stressors, such as a demanding job, young children, a very strict budget, and little to no support. That's why there's no one-size-fits-all answer as to what number of changes is too much or not enough.

However, there is a guideline you can adhere to and apply to your individual life so you can do the best you can with what you have and without stressing out so much you break out in hives: Reduce (not eliminate) toxins in your environment as much as you can. But when you find yourself at the place where reducing your *toxin* burden is increasing your *stress* burden, that's a sign that it may be becoming more harmful than helpful and you need to apply the brakes. And, at least in this season of your life, that is okay.

I'm more than five years into my cleaner-living journey and have not yet overhauled my whole wardrobe or every textile in my home (which, surprise, surprise, apparently have harmful toxins too). I've invested in air filters and water filters as well as made some swaps, including our cookware, our mattresses, and a few pieces in my closet. But the thought of getting rid of all my favorite clothes and changing out all our furniture is stressful and overwhelming, so I am taking my sweet time with it, making a little shift here and there so as not to throw myself into a frenzy.

> When you find yourself at the place where reducing your *toxin* burden is increasing your *stress* burden, that's a sign that it may be becoming more harmful than helpful.

BEING GOOD TO YOUR BODY IS LIGHTENING YOUR LOAD

There's a scripture I love and often come back to when I feel as though I'm beginning to teeter on the line between obedience and obsession, or stewardship and stress. In Matthew 11:28–30, there's an invitation from Jesus: "Come to me, all who labor and are heavy laden, and I will give you rest. Take my yoke upon you, and learn from me, for I am gentle and lowly in heart, and you will find rest for your souls. For my yoke is easy, and my burden is light."

The truth is, both toxins and stress are burdens on our bodies, but Jesus offers us a better way. His yoke is *easy* and His burden is *light*. Caring for our bodies biblically, as a response to God and from a place of obedience and stewardship, should not feel exhausting, stressful, or burdensome. Instead, it should feel intentional, life-giving, and light.

In order to do that, we must invite Jesus into every moment of our journeys. We can't pursue health or healing on our own. We just can't. We have sinful hearts that tend toward either obsession or apathy, and we desperately need supernatural wisdom and guidance for each decision we make.

That is where I got off track at one point (and can easily get off track again if I'm not careful). The problem wasn't that I was trying to make healthier choices; it's that I was trying to make healthier choices without inviting God into those decisions or allowing Him to guide me through them. And as a result, I was putting my hope in healthy things and in healing my body all on my own, which is a heavy burden none of us is meant to bear.

It became so much less stressful when I began to be more prayerful and looked to the creator of my body to show me which changes I was called to make or disciplines I needed to implement. I started asking the Lord to help me see which of the random information I come across online is *for* me and what is *not* for me, to honor and bless the ways I'm trying to support my body, and to remind me of His sovereignty over all that I can't control or that could harm me.

I didn't suddenly stop supporting my health and well-being in the name of avoiding all stress, but I did gain more clarity on which swaps, steps, and disciplines needed to be priorities for me at a given time (and which did not). That helped my pursuit of health become more peaceful instead of frantic and stressful.

So, what's my point? Being good to your body involves accepting Jesus's invitation. It's reducing your toxins, which, yes, are a type of body burden. But it's also releasing the weight of carrying burdens you were never meant to carry yourself, and that is done by allowing God to direct your pursuit of health.

When we partner with God in anything, the burden becomes lighter. Although the journey may not be easy, it is less heavy. Instead of trying to be in the driver's seat—or being the gods of our lives—we allow God to be in His rightful place and we follow *His* lead.

Obsession and stress result from believing the lie the Enemy whispers to us that we are on our own and everything is on our shoulders. That's a heavy load to carry, and it's one we were never meant to bear. But obedience and stewardship result from believing the truth that although our disciplines and decisions *do* hold weight, we have a good Father who is ultimately sovereign over every little thing.

That is the light burden Jesus was talking about and invites us into.

And to me, in a world that's full of enough pressure to perform, trends to keep up with, and to-dos, that is good news.

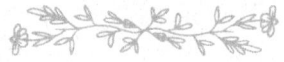

PRAYER

God, I pray for a peaceful heart, a clear mind, and a steadfast spirit. I ask for protection from all the pollutants and toxins in my environment that I cannot control or remove at this time, and for wisdom over the proactive changes I can make. Show me which swaps are mine to own and what I need to set down or stop stressing about for now. Amen.

PRACTICAL APPLICATION

Consider your toxin burden, including stress (which is a toxin). Where could you lighten your load? Are there a few products you could afford to swap out? Is it possibly time to invest in a good water filter? What is one way you can support your body's detoxification? Can you implement a daily workout routine that will get you sweating? Or maybe work on staying hydrated? Do a weekly castor oil pack for your liver? Reduce sugar? Something else? Or are you at capacity with swapping and stressing about everything and instead need to invite God on the journey, leaning on His sovereignty (instead of your own)? Take some time to think about that and then make one fruitful change, whether in your environment or your mindset.

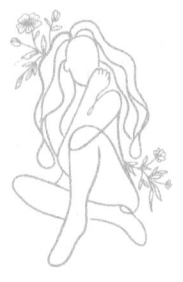

Chapter 9

RECLAIM YOUR FEMININITY

Throughout my fertility and subsequent wellness journey, I ran the gamut of testing, including a DUTCH test. No, that's not a test to see if I have any Dutch heritage, although that *would* be cool. It stands for Dried Urine Test for Comprehensive Hormones.

Did I seriously just tell you I had my dried pee tested? Yes. Yes, I did.

Maybe it's TMI and slightly embarrassing, but I'm sharing for a reason, so just hang with me. I did this test per the recommendation of a hormone specialist I was working with when I told her I hadn't been sleeping well. I had trouble falling asleep at night and would often wake up not feeling rested in the morning.

We opted for a DUTCH test to get a more comprehensive picture of how my hormones were behaving because it tests over the course of a twenty-four-hour period as opposed to a blood test that captures data at only one moment in time. Without getting into all the nitty-gritty details, basically the DUTCH test evaluates metabolites and biomarkers derived from estrogens, progesterone, and androgens. Additionally, it gives a complete look at cortisol (stress hormone) in the body.

> Free cortisol is the active form of the hormone which binds to receptors and turns them on. Testing free cortisol helps understand the circadian rhythm and answers questions about a patient's low energy and sleep trouble.
>
> DUTCH . . . includes . . . cortisol because it can be influenced by stress and more.[1]

So, anyway, I sent in my dry urine samples and awaited the results. Once they were in, I met with my healthcare provider to go over everything. We talked through my estrogen, progesterone, and various other levels, and then we got to the cortisol section. It was displayed as a little chart. My cortisol line on the graph was nearly flat. It didn't spike. In fact, there wasn't much of a curve at all.

I was genuinely surprised to see that. I mean, I *felt* stressed, but it seemed like my results were showing otherwise.

"Oh good!" I exclaimed with relief. "I'm not as stressed as I thought!"

My provider looked at me for a moment. "No," she said, "that's not what this means."

Puzzled, I asked her to go on.

"You *should* have a healthy curve when it comes to cortisol. Yes, it's the stress hormone, and *too much* isn't good. But your body needs a healthy amount of cortisol for energy and normal functioning. It should rise to a healthy place in the morning and then slowly decrease throughout the rest of the day. This tells me you've been operating with chronically elevated cortisol levels for so long that your adrenals are basically shot and now your body can barely produce the needed and healthy levels of cortisol for natural energy. Sometimes this is referred to as adrenal fatigue."

She went on to explain that the adrenal glands are small organs that sit on top of the kidneys and produce hormones that regulate such things as metabolism, blood pressure, and the immune system. You know, nothing too important.

It was, in fact, worse than I thought. *Fabulous.*

"So what do I do about it?" I asked.

Before answering my question, my provider asked about my lifestyle, schedule, and sleep and how well I was supporting my circadian and infradian rhythms.

As a refresher, an infradian rhythm is a biological cycle that lasts longer than twenty-four hours. Examples in nature include things like hibernation, migration, breeding, and molting. In women, the menstrual cycle is an infradian rhythm, and it can affect a woman's health in many ways.[2]

Anyway, I walked her through a typical day of mine: I'd wake up, drink coffee, do some sort of intense-cardio workout, get ready for the day, work until I got hungry, eat a salad or pick up something quick for lunch, continue working, have more coffee, make dinner, clean up, and then scroll on my phone or watch a show until I went to bed. I told her how it took me forever to fall asleep. I just felt wired at night and couldn't shut my brain off. And then in the morning, I felt like I was dragging. It was as if when I needed energy and when I needed to wind down were reversed.

She explained how the habits and rhythms I had in my life weren't supporting my internal clock or biological needs and how some simple shifts could support my adrenal health, which would help restore my body's circadian rhythm, natural energy, sleep, and overall well-being.

Here are some of the tweaks she suggested:

- Cut back on caffeine, and if I did drink coffee, try to choose an organic option and only consume it with a protein-rich breakfast instead of on an empty stomach.
- Try mixing up workouts with strength training instead of doing only intense cardio, and include gentler movement more often, such as Pilates and walking.
- Get an old-school alarm clock instead of sleeping near my cell phone.
- Shut all screens and blue-light devices off one hour before going to bed.
- Eat a nourishing snack thirty to sixty minutes before bed to keep blood sugar stable.
- Set an earlier bedtime and try to go to bed around the same time every night and wake up around the same time every morning.
- Get sunlight first thing in the morning, before looking at a screen.
- Drink an adrenal mocktail daily to support minerals and adrenal health with essentials like sodium, potassium, and vitamin C.
- Slow down and set some boundaries on work and extra commitments; allow myself to be bored, read a book, and have white space on my calendar.

I was a little skeptical but took her advice. I focused on supporting my sleep, tried to prioritize nourishing food over caffeine for energy, shifted to gentler workouts, and cut back on screen time by opting to read books before bed instead of watching a show or scrolling on my phone.

Within a couple of months, my energy improved significantly. I was sleeping better, my moods stabilized, I snapped at my husband less, and I felt more like me again.

The breakneck speed at which I had been living and trying to achieve things was really a more masculine, rather than feminine, way of doing things. Hustle, doing the same thing every day, intense cardio—all those things may be suitable to the masculine physiology but can be stressors on the feminine body. By resisting hustle, slowing down, and tuning in to my biological needs, I was able to lean back into my God-given femininity.

> Hustle, doing the same thing every day, intense cardio—all those things may be suitable to the masculine physiology but can be stressors on the feminine body.

And in the process, I experienced not just adrenal recovery but also a deeper healing—a reclaiming of a part of me I didn't even know I had lost or realize I needed.

THE FEMININE URGE TO SLOW DOWN

I didn't need a fancy test to know I needed to change some things. It was obvious by my lack of energy, struggle to sleep well, and general sense of overwhelm and anxiety. How I was operating was clearly not serving me or my body's needs.

But sometimes it helps to see the facts plainly. And once I saw the science behind what I was feeling, I knew it was time to listen to that urge I had been having to slow down.

My friend Annika says it beautifully: "The feminine urge to slow down is a biological need, not laziness or a lack of ambition."

I don't know about you, but I need that reminder *daily*.

Whether we're professionals building our careers, students staying up late studying, or stay-at-home-moms running kids here and there and everywhere, all of us can get caught up in the societal norm of busyness, overcommitment, and fast-paced living. In other words, it's not just a girl-boss thing; it's *normal* in our culture for women to be overly busy and burned-out.

In fact, a 2018 Gallup poll found that millennials are more likely than other generations to be burned-out,[3] and in a LinkedIn survey of almost five thousand Americans, 74 percent of the women said they were somewhat or very stressed because of work, compared with 61 percent of the men.[4] Translation of these two facts combined: Millennial women may be one of the most stressed and burned-out demographics. Perhaps it's because we've settled for what's normal. But just because something is *normal* doesn't mean it is *beneficial.*

> The feminine urge to slow down is a biological need, not laziness or a lack of ambition.
> —Annika

What's normal? Chronic busyness, living on caffeine and convenience food, running in a hundred directions, trying to "do it all" between building big careers and taking on a majority share of home responsibilities, and existing in a constant state of stress. And the "normal" solution to that stress is usually some kind of quick fix, whether that's a spa day, a mind-numbing distraction (such as social media or Netflix), taking a vacation, or even turning to substances (ever heard of "mommy wine culture"?).

Even though taking a nap, getting a massage, eating dinner with friends, or going on vacation can be great ways to recharge, those do not necessarily equate to slowing down. Instead, truly slowing down involves creating a *lifestyle* with regular rhythms of rest and establishing habits that allow us to support our God-given design and biological needs.

As we've discussed, women are cyclical beings, with infradian rhythms, so doing the same thing day in and day out, hustling hard with stressful deadlines, and living within the confines of the nine-to-five grind does not support our bodies' natural needs. In its most pure form, the feminine nature is more creative, slow, and relational.

If you look at the hormone cycles of males and females, they are entirely different. Some hormone educators I've interviewed or learned from explain it like this: "Women are like the moon and men are like the sun."[5] Women's hormone cycles follow that infradian rhythm over the course of a month, whereas men's hormone cycles follow the twenty-four-hour cycle, which aligns with the circadian rhythm. That is why the grind suits them well and they're able to get up, work out, clock in, and do a lot of the same things day in and day out.

Notice I said "hormone cycles." What does that even mean? Here's a quick breakdown regarding men:[6]

- In the morning, men's testosterone levels are high, which can make them feel energized, focused, and ready to work.
- Later in the afternoon, testosterone levels drop some, which can make men feel more social and ready to connect with other people.
- Then, into the evening, their testosterone levels continue to decrease, which can make them want to relax.

How is that different for women?[7]

- We have four phases of our twenty-eight-ish-day hormone cycle: menstrual, follicular, ovulatory, and luteal.
- In the menstrual phase ("the period"), there is a hormone drop so that the uterine lining can shed. At that time, we

are generally lower on energy and need more rest. (The body is bleeding for days at a time, so that only makes sense.)

- In the follicular phase, estrogen and progesterone levels are low and then begin to increase steadily as a follicle develops and produces more estrogen. As estrogen increases, we are most likely to have new ideas, feel more creative, and plan ahead.
- Then, in the ovulatory phase, which is generally a few days around the middle of our cycles, we have a spike in testosterone, which can make us feel more social and energized (similar to a man in the afternoon of his twenty-four-hour cycle).
- After ovulation and before the next period is the luteal phase. Progesterone levels increase for up to eight days after ovulation. If an egg is not fertilized, progesterone levels begin to drop until the uterine lining begins to shed, which marks the start of a new cycle, beginning with menstruation. During the luteal phase, we are likely to feel our most focused, productive, and organized (at least more so than at other times of our cycles).

Clearly, the female hormone cycle has little to no resemblance to the male hormone cycle on a daily basis. Our energy is not the same day to day or even week to week, and that is important to understand as we make our plans and create rhythms and routines that support our bodies.[8]

I know that was a whole science lesson you didn't ask for, but I share it because once I began to understand how my female body was actually designed to work, I was able to see where certain routines, habits, and societal norms I just thought I was "supposed to do" (get up at 5 A.M. to work out every day, work nine to five Monday through Friday, and so on) may not actually be very supportive to my feminine physiology. And I realized that maybe the lack of motivation or energy I had at different times of the month was not actually laziness but instead my body expressing the need for a slower pace because of all that it was doing.

Anyway, that is based on my own understanding and experience in learning from various research and hormone experts, but the science behind the difference in female and male hormones alone backs up what the Bible tells us about our design.

Genesis 1:27 says that God, in His infinite wisdom, made us different from men: "God created man in his own image . . . *male* and *female* he created them" (emphasis added).

Not better or worse, just *different*.

Ignoring that to keep up with societal norms and the pressure to hustle, achieve, please everyone, say yes to everything, or break glass ceilings isn't serving our biological needs or physiological well-being. Does that mean we shouldn't work? Of course not.

But it does mean we may need to work and achieve at a different pace. That is biblical and critical as we seek to be good to our bodies.

BEING GOOD TO YOUR BODY IS SLOWING DOWN AND SUPPORTING YOUR FEMININE PHYSIOLOGY

The real and sustainable solution to our fast-paced living, stress and burnout, and subsequent health problems is found in the example and invitation to rest that God laid out for us in the very first few pages of the Bible: slowing down and creating simple rhythms that support our bodies *and our souls* so we can live aligned with how He designed us to thrive.

Genesis 2:2 tells us that God rested on the seventh day of creation. And in Mark 2:27, Jesus said, "The Sabbath was made for man, not man for the Sabbath." That is, Sabbath rest—regular, rhythmic rest—is a divine institution, a gift *for* us, that benefits both our souls and bodies.

We are made in His image, which means we need to rest rhythmically and regularly. Despite living in a society that makes rest out to be a quick self-care splurge, slowing down isn't a luxury; it is fundamental to our well-being and to meeting our most basic needs.

Furthermore, in Genesis 2:15, we find that God put man in the garden to tend to it and keep it. We are called to tend to and steward creation. As I've already stated, our bodies are part of that creation. If we are designed for rest, we *must* give that to our bodies (as well as to our hearts and minds) in order to obey the command to steward creation well.

Let's look at this verse literally. If you've ever had an actual garden, you know it's a slow process. It requires you to stop, tend, weed, water, and nourish for it to flourish. And guess what? The same is true for us. Stewardship cannot happen when we're stressed-out and running a million miles an hour, because when we're moving too fast, it's hard to see what needs attention—what needs tending. It requires that we slow down, notice what needs support, and nourish our bodies well.

This might look like making the kinds of simple lifestyle shifts my provider recommended when my adrenals were shot: unplugging from devices by a certain time, setting boundaries on our availability, moving our bodies a little more gently, prioritizing prayer before productivity, and getting sunlight into our eyes before looking at a screen in the morning.

Lastly, remember that Genesis 2:18 tells us that God said, "It is not good for the man to be alone. I will make a helper suitable for him" (NIV). Fundamentally, that means that God, who created human beings, believes community is a good thing. And being good to our bodies means giving them the good things God created for us, right? Creating rhythms where we disconnect from devices, take a pause in our productivity, and spend time with the ones we love is a necessity for our well-being.

Being good to your body requires a slower way of living. But remember that slowing down doesn't just mean resting and relaxing randomly or neglecting your work or God-given duties; it means creating rhythms and habits that allow you to support your feminine physiology, rest your mind and your body, and live a little more aligned with your God-given design, one day at a time.

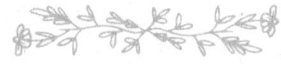

PRAYER

God, thank You for my feminine body. Help me embrace and celebrate what makes it unique and remind me that my need for rest does not make me lazy or weak. I want to learn to overcome the pressure to function at a nonstop, breakneck speed just because it's normal to be busy. I know that hustle and burnout are not from You and that You are a God of peace and are never in a hurry. Help me be more like that. Show me where I can slow down, be still, and implement some simple habits and routines into my lifestyle to support my body and live a little more aligned with Your good and perfect design. Amen.

PRACTICAL APPLICATION

This week, try one of these ways to slow down. Then see if you can incorporate more ways into your life over the weeks and months to come.

- *Read books instead of scrolling social media or watching TV the last thirty minutes before bed.*
- *Spend time in the Bible and prayer before work.*
- *Leave your phone in another room for extended periods of time and ideally turn it off at least one hour before going to bed and wait to look at it until one hour after you wake up.*
- *Go to bed by 10:00 P.M. and wake up early to have time to yourself (unless you're up all night with babies, in which case you have a pass here for a season).*
- *Learn the phases of your cycle and consider how you might shift your workouts, professional projects, and social plans to support your body's energy and biological needs more naturally.*
- *Find a recipe you really love—maybe a fancy dinner, a tasty dessert—and pick one weekend a month where you'll put your phone away, turn on some happy music, and make the recipe at home.*
- *Go for walks after dinner.*

- *Open your window or step outside in the morning to get sunlight.*
- *Create a regular Sabbath where you unplug from work, social media, and extracurricular obligations one day per week or month with your family.*

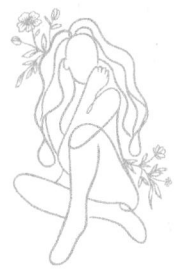

Chapter 10

EMBRACE YOUR BEAUTY *NATURALLY*

I looked in the mirror and felt the furthest thing from beautiful. I saw tired eyes from sleep deprivation, some thin patches of hair on the side of my head thanks to postpartum hair loss, a fresh new pimple on my chin, a squishier middle than I'd ever had before, loose skin, and a brand-new scar from a natural-birth plan turned unexpected C-section.

I splashed water on my face and stepped back for a moment. As I did, I was reminded what my mom once taught me about beauty when I didn't feel my prettiest after a miscarriage years earlier. She had said, "As our hearts and bodies go through trials, it helps us understand how strong and beautiful our bodies are as we see them weather that storm. You're losing ease and gaining depth. And that's beauty—a different type of beauty. A deeper beauty. Now you have a little 'patina.'"

I asked what *patina* means. Patina is essentially when something appears to have grown more beautiful with time or age. In the literal sense, it might be thought of as that green film that naturally forms on materials like copper and bronze. Over time, as the surface of the materials is exposed or worn, they gain patina, which is often regarded as beautiful and valued aesthetically.

Every time I've doubted my body's strength or beauty since that day, I'm reminded that patina is beautiful—that when I look in the mirror and see tired eyes, scars, or other reminders of the battles I've fought and the life my body has lived, I should try to remember they don't take away from my beauty—they add to it. Those are marks of the hard-won depth, wisdom, and character I've gained—my patina. And I don't know about you, but I'll gladly trade simply looking pretty for a worn, deep, inner beauty that doesn't fade.

As I reflected on that conversation with my mom while staring at my disheveled appearance in the mirror, I realized that maybe it wasn't so much that I didn't see *beauty* but that I just didn't feel very *pretty*.

What do you think? Is there a difference?

I think so. We may use these words interchangeably, but *pretty* is often used to describe a pleasing outward appearance—pleasing to the eye. *Beautiful* is deeper than that, where something is pleasing to not only the eye but also the senses and mind.

In other words, "pretty" is surface level. And while "beautiful" may include appearance, it is more than skin-deep. True beauty begins in the heart and mind. It's wisdom, selflessness, and emotional intelligence. A beautiful woman does not clamor to be seen. She is quick to listen and slow to speak. She's thoughtful and courageous. She speaks truth in love, exudes kindness, and walks in integrity.

If I asked you to think of a beautiful woman you know, who comes to mind? At first you may think of an old college roommate, a friend, or a particular influencer you follow online—the one with amazing hair, flawless skin, and other enviable features. But if you think about who embodies the characteristics of a truly beautiful woman, I'd be willing to bet someone else comes to mind. She may not be a size 2 or keep up on the latest fashion trends, she may have salt-and-pepper hair or deep smile lines, but she probably *also* has wisdom, a selfless heart, a warm smile, a gentle courage, and tender strength.

> Anyone can *look pretty*, but it takes a special kind of woman to *be beautiful*.

Maybe it's your grandma, your mom, your mentor, or a friend you think of as an older sister. Maybe it's someone you connected with through work or church. Maybe it's the local coffee shop owner who has kind eyes, knows you by name, and offers a warm smile as she asks thoughtful questions about your life whenever she takes your order. You may not be very close with her personally, but she makes you feel cared for and seen with her intentionality.

Why am I so set on highlighting the contrast between these two words? Well, with a little work, anyone can *look pretty*, but it takes a special kind of woman to *be beautiful*.

Whether through harsh treatments, toxic injections, or invasive procedures, the world offers countless ways to squeeze, tuck, fill, and manipulate the body in unnatural ways. Many women are so quickly opting in to it, chasing after looking *pretty*, that they don't even realize that what they're really after is *beauty*—a beauty that transcends the physical and cultural standards we are bombarded with daily.

> True beauty cannot be achieved by focusing on the body or appearance alone.

And true beauty cannot be achieved by focusing on the body or appearance alone. But does that mean that our bodies and appearance don't matter? Far from it. They matter more than we think, and how we care for them speaks volumes about the beliefs we hold about our maker and the work of His hands.

BEAUTY IS IMPORTANT, BUT IT ISN'T ULTIMATE

I know we've discussed this already, but it's relevant here. If we go back to the very beginning of the Bible, in the Creation account, Genesis 1:27 tells us that our creator made us in His image. And just a bit later in Genesis 2:15, we see that man was placed in the garden with the responsibility, or duty, to tend to and care for creation.

Some say that the beauty of creation is a reminder of God and that respecting His creation shows value for what He has created and admiration for the Creator. I couldn't agree more. The truth is, *we* are part of that creation, and how we care for our bodies and beauty directly reflects how we respect and value God's creation.

> How we care for our bodies and beauty directly reflects how we respect and value God's creation.

If we believe we are made in His image and agree that our bodies are a divine, God-given gift, then it doesn't make logical sense to neglect any part of it, including our hair, our skin, or anything else that might fall under the category of "beauty."

It is my firm conviction that Christian women have spent far too long believing the lie that it is somehow holy to neglect any part of physical beauty because all that matters is the spiritual. When I look at the Bible, that line of thinking just misses the mark. It's *close* to the truth in that physical appearance is not ultimate and that what matters most is the heart, but it's not the whole story.

For example, Proverbs 31:30 says that "charm is deceptive, and beauty is fleeting" (NIV), and I believe that wholeheartedly. But if we look at the whole description of a virtuous woman, we find that she *also* clothed herself in scarlet (a very nice material) and worked to make her arms strong (took care of her body) (see verses 21, 17).

Furthermore, the apostle Peter wrote, "Your beauty should not come from outward adornment, such as elaborate hairstyles and the wearing of gold jewelry or fine clothes. Rather, it should be that of your inner self, the unfading beauty of a gentle and quiet spirit, which is of great worth in God's sight" (1 Peter 3:3–4, NIV).

So, does that mean we throw out all our accessories and forget about physical appearance and beauty entirely? Not at all. It simply means we do not make outward appearance our main source of beauty.

I think of Queen Esther here. Before being considered by the king, she completed a yearlong period of beauty treatments. *A whole year.* The Bible says, "Before a young woman's turn came to go in to King Xerxes, she had to complete twelve months of beauty treatments prescribed for the women" (Esther 2:12, NIV).

Those treatments, while extensive, were meant to *enhance* her natural beauty and *optimize* the health of her physical features (such as her hair and skin), not manipulate or change them altogether. While Esther's outward appearance likely helped her gain the king's favor, she also displayed humility and character, which some scholars believe may have helped her stand out among the other candidates and win over the king and all who saw her.

True beauty is found in character, not just physical appearance. But that doesn't mean physical beauty is of no importance, because if you truly believe you are made in the image of God—that you are fearfully and wonderfully made—you understand that your body is sacred and to be cared for. Yes, that can and does look like working out and eating well. But let's not forget that your body also includes your face and hair, and it is simply good stewardship to care for the health of those things too. The idea that it's more holy to neglect those things makes zero sense if we're looking at a holistic view of the body as a sacred vessel, our creator's workmanship, and a gift.

Does that mean you *have* to wear makeup, style your hair, and get regular facials? Of course not. But it does mean there should not be shame in caring for the physical appearance, as if the physical is not sacred.

A godly woman understands that beauty is fleeting and that a fear of the Lord is to be praised—that it is the mark of true beauty. So she doesn't put her hope or trust in her outward appearance but *does* understand that her physical body and appearance are sacred gifts and that caring for, maintaining, or enhancing them naturally is not inherently ungodly.

True beauty cannot be achieved with physical appearance alone, but it also cannot be achieved by neglecting it under the guise of holiness.

Keeping the right perspective with a humble-heart posture can help us maintain and care for our outward appearance in response to God instead of making it a god itself.

Perhaps one of the most devastating things I learned on my health journey was how little regulation there is in the beauty industry and, as a result, the large amount of harmful ingredients women are being exposed to every day just in the time that they get ready in the morning.

According to the Environmental Working Group (EWG), the average woman uses twelve products per day, putting approximately 168 potentially harmful chemicals on her body just in her hygiene and beauty routines.[1] That doesn't even include all the other environmental toxins she may be exposed to in her water, air, textiles, and household products.

Just beauty.

Our society is riddled with toxic beauty products, extreme treatments, and invasive procedures. These days, it's just considered normal to get lip filler and Botox injections. And if that's you, I'm not here to shame you, but I do want us to consider how widespread it is and whether those types of things are actually good for our bodies.

It's one thing to wear makeup, especially if that makeup is not laden with countless toxins linked to countless health concerns, but it's another to lather on or even inject toxic ingredients into the body in the name of beauty.

Corporations capitalize on our insecurities and sell us the promise of being skinnier, prettier, and more confident—even if their products, treatments, and procedures are quite literally toxic to human cells and harmful to the body. To top it off, it's often all wrapped up in women-empowerment language.

But is it truly *pro-woman* if it's harmful to women's health? I mean, what's empowering about that? In one way or another, we've all fallen for it, from toxic products all the way to implants and Botox.

Let me pause and say: zero judgment and no shame if you've chosen any of those things. To some degree, most of us have. But there has to be a better way.

A BIBLICAL TAKE ON BEAUTY

If we look at Genesis, we find that beauty is a theme throughout it. That book of the Bible highlights the beauty of God's creation, humanity, and divinity.

Romans 1:20 states, "Since the creation of the world God's invisible qualities—his eternal power and divine nature—have been clearly seen, being understood from what has been made" (NIV).

In other words, beauty matters to God. He created beautiful things that reveal His character and power. We are made in His image and, by nature, are creative. It makes sense that we also care about beauty. We mimic our creator by creating beautiful things, including tasteful hairstyles, makeup looks, or even outfits that accompany a God-fearing heart. That is a *good* thing.

Remember, 1 Peter 3:3–4 tells us that inner beauty is more important than outward appearance. Outward appearance *does* matter to an extent. We should do what we can to maintain or enhance it. But, ultimately, it doesn't matter how pretty someone looks, because if they are selfish, greedy, unkind, or dishonest, they do not have beauty. To be attractive on the outside but lack the inner beauty that comes from faith in God is a burden more than it is a blessing.

The Bible supports, and is the basis for, the argument that beauty is more than skin-deep.

BACK TO BEAUTY

As a reminder, stewardship is how we behave and what we choose when we believe, "Everything I have is Yours, God."

It's easy to inject, twist, tuck, and manipulate our bodies if we view them as our own, with no accountability about what we do to them or put into or on them. It's not so easy when we view our bodies—every detail of them, including our outward appearance—as the Lord's.

If you remember back in chapter 1, I shared the metaphor of borrowing a car from a friend. I would do my best to maintain and care for the car, right? It would be reasonable to get it washed, clean the inside, and get the tires rotated if I were driving it long distances or borrowing it for an extended time. It would not be so reasonable for me to go crazy and paint the car an entirely different color, outrageously customize the wheels, install a fancy speaker system, or do anything else to it that would drastically change its appearance.

Why? Because it's not mine to re-create with expensive, extreme measures that make the car unrecognizable. And it's not that different with our bodies.

Fillers, fake teeth (veneers), breast implants, and the like are common in our culture. But I often say that just because something is common does not mean it is *good* for us.

BEING GOOD TO YOUR BODY IS
A RETURN TO HOLISTIC BEAUTY

I mentioned Esther's yearlong beauty regimen, and I thought it might be worth taking a closer look at it and seeing what wisdom we might glean from it. Let's again look at Esther 2:12: "Before a young woman's turn came to go in to King Xerxes, she had to complete twelve months of beauty treatments prescribed for the women, six months with oil of myrrh and six with perfumes and cosmetics" (NIV).

While we don't know all the exact details of her treatments, we can gain some insight by considering what beauty treatments typically entailed at that time of biblical history: oils, myrrh, honey, milk baths, botanicals, cosmetics, clay, and floral hydrosols. Do you notice what's common to all these beauty treatments? They are from the earth—they are natural, with mechanisms for healing, health, and radiance.

For example, myrrh is a medicinal plant and believed to have anti-microbial and anti-inflammatory properties. It has been reported to stimulate circulation, decrease inflammation, soothe inflamed skin, heal fungal infections, and more.[2] Olive oil has antioxidant and anti-inflammatory qualities. It has been linked to improved skin hydration as well as anti-aging effects.[3] And honey is a natural moisturizer. It retains moisture, is mildly antiseptic, and has anti-inflammatory properties that have been found to be helpful for skin conditions such as acne.[4]

Esther's beauty treatments may have been extensive, but they were natural, not disruptive to hormones or invasive to the body, and ultimately designed to improve her well-being and enhance her natural beauty, not manipulate or change her appearance altogether.

Whoa, how far have we come from that? Modern treatments are hardly natural at all anymore unless you really seek them out.

What if being good to our bodies looked like turning to nature and natural ingredients more than we turn to invasive procedures and toxic cosmetics? What if our approach to beauty was more holistic and aligned with God's design? What if caring for our outward appearance was *more* than simply using foundation or getting fillers? What if it instead began with what we do or use daily: the food we eat, the personal-care products we use, how we sleep, and the ways we care for our bodies?

How powerful would that be, and how much healthier would we feel? How much more radiant would our skin be if we cared for our appearance from the inside out and prioritized natural treatments over toxic products or invasive procedures that come with countless side effects?

That's not to say throw out all your beauty products, never wear makeup, or give up on ever getting a manicure. It's just to say that maybe it's time we take a bit more of a natural, countercultural, inside-out (instead of merely a topical or quick-fix) approach.

Maybe Queen Esther teaches us a thing or two about being good to our bodies in how we approach beauty. Maybe part of being good to our bodies is getting back to nature and understanding that what we put in and on our bodies should be done thoughtfully and that it may be wise to prioritize more on natural beauty treatments (serums, moisturizers, cosmetics, perfumes) than on procedures and products full of hormone disruptors, heavy metals, and known carcinogens that may do more harm than good.

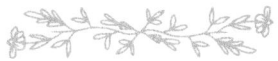

PRAYER

God, thank You for creating beautiful things and for the body You gave me. I know beauty matters to You and that You have "made everything beautiful in its time" (Ecclesiastes 3:11). Help me learn to embrace my features and enhance my natural beauty instead of trying to completely change my appearance to look like a copy-and-paste of someone else. I confess that I have felt envy toward others I believe are prettier than me and I have been guilty of chasing after looking pretty because I've believed culture's definitions of beauty instead of Scripture's. Forgive me, Lord, and help me focus on true beauty in a world obsessed with looking pretty. Amen.

PRACTICAL APPLICATION

Consider the ways you can focus on building a healthier beauty routine. Here are some ideas:

- *Check the labels on the beauty products you're using regularly and replace any that have harmful ingredients with safer options. (You can use my label-reading cheat sheet located at the back of this book to make it easier to check for the main ingredients I try to avoid.)*
- *Focus on nourishment and prioritize real, nutrient-dense food as much as possible. For example, things like collagen (found in bone broth), carrots, and grass-fed gelatin (make some gummies!) can be great for hair and skin health.*
- *Spend time in the sun—natural vitamin D!*
- *Create a bedtime routine you can stick with to support quality sleep.*
- *Find ways to incorporate Scripture into your daily routine. (I love listening to The Bible Recap podcast while making my kids breakfast!)*
- *Hydrate to support cellular and metabolic health from the inside out.*
- *Try dry brushing for lymphatic support before taking a shower.*

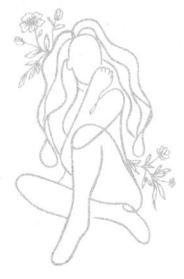

Chapter 11

SUPPORT YOUR FERTILITY

I got on birth control when I was twenty-two. My wedding was approaching and I was a virgin. So when I told my ob-gyn that I wasn't ready to even think about getting pregnant (and kind of hoped I could avoid being on my period for my wedding), she quickly scribbled me a script for birth control and sent me on my way.

We had no conversations about understanding my body or natural ways to avoid pregnancy—just a prescription for pills that the World Health Organization (WHO) has named a class-one carcinogen, mind you.[1]

But I didn't ask questions. I just went and filled the script without thinking twice about it. I mean, I wanted to be a mom *eventually* but had just graduated from college and had goals I wanted to achieve first. I was young, practically a baby myself. I couldn't possibly risk having a baby (even though I would be married).

Oh how I wish I could go back and tell my younger self what I know now.

Thankfully, I took the pill for less than a year before something inside me thought, *Hmm, maybe this isn't something I want to be on long-term.*

However, perhaps not so coincidentally, when I stopped taking birth control, my skin broke out in cystic acne, my hormones were a mess, and it was as if my body began to revolt against me. And I hadn't even been on it that long! Then, as you already know, once I decided I was ready to have a baby a few years later, I unexpectedly struggled with pregnancy loss and trying to get pregnant, and I began to regret ever suppressing my fertility in the first place.

I think we've been sold a lie, and it's come at a high cost. It's become quite common for women to use toxic chemicals and synthetic hormones to suppress fertility during their peak childbearing years to either relieve unwanted symptoms (such as irregular periods or acne) or avoid becoming pregnant, under the assumption that a baby will just come easily if and when they decide they are "ready."

Nancy Pearcey, in her book *Love Thy Body*, references the words of economist Jennifer Roback Morse, who spoke from her own experience in regard to this subject: "Here is the bargain we professional women have been making. . . . To achieve higher levels of education and professionalism, women are required to suppress their fertility with birth control—to neuter themselves with toxic chemicals during their peak childbearing."[2]

Morse concluded that young women "are being sold a cynical lie," because they have accepted the cultural expectation that they must get established in a career before they can think seriously about starting a family. "They do not realize they are giving themselves over to careers during their peak fertility years, with the expectation that somehow, someday, they can 'have it all.'"[3]

Pearcey concludes: "The problem is that when women are finally established in their careers, many are finding that their fertility has declined . . . and they are no longer able to have the families they want. At that point, they are subjecting themselves to invasive, expensive, and often disappointing fertility treatments."[4]

Wow. They're not wrong, but that is tough to digest, especially as Western women who are blessed to have the opportunities we do.

Maybe, like I was, you've been put on birth control without being told about your options or without anyone explaining the potential risks. Maybe this is the first time you've ever heard there could be risks or thought twice about it. And I get it. I've been there. It is well marketed not only as a way to avoid pregnancy but also as a quick fix (otherwise known as a Band-Aid) for various symptoms women often face.

Understandably, no one wants to deal with symptoms a simple little pill can seemingly relieve, and no one wants to be irresponsible by getting pregnant without being able to provide for a baby or jumping into parenthood before they're ready. But at the same time, where is the line? Is it worth the potential risks and side effects?

I used to believe that I could control the timing of pregnancy and that once I felt I had achieved enough professionally and was *ready* (whatever that means—I mean, do you ever really feel totally ready?), it would just happen. But then it didn't. And as we struggled through multiple years of recurrent miscarriages and even a bout of infertility, I wished I could have gone back and told my younger self not to artificially suppress my fertility in the first place.

I realized in those years of struggling to have a family that there is a much healthier and more sustainable way to address unwanted symptoms. I also realized that business and professional goals and money would always be there—that they were things I could come back to or put more energy and time into building down the road—but my childbearing years would not.

And, unfortunately, it's often not until we walk through something like infertility that we come to understand that reality. I had to come face-to-face with the fact that just because you decide you're ready to have a family doesn't mean it'll be easy to get pregnant (and that even a positive test doesn't always lead to bringing home a baby). And now I wish I could tell every woman not to believe the lie that she should suppress her fertility and risk sacrificing her desired future family at the altar of money or success or quick fixes just because that's become normal in our society.

Now, please hear me. I'm not saying a woman has to get married and have a baby to live a full life or be happy. That's not necessarily every woman's calling or desire. Here's what I *am* saying: There's nothing wrong with working. It's great for a woman to be able to financially provide for herself or do what she loves. I'm all about that. But suppressing symptoms and fertility with hormonal birth control that WHO has named a carcinogen? That just cannot be good for our bodies.

THE LINK BETWEEN FERTILITY, FEMININITY, AND IDENTITY

"Maybe it was just a bad egg," my ob-gyn said with a shrug as I asked question after question, desperate to understand what went wrong after my first miscarriage.

A bad egg? I wondered. *Do I have bad eggs? Is this my fault?*

Her answer was probably pretty standard from a medical perspective. She saw that kind of thing frequently, and it wasn't personal for her like it was for me. Plus, she didn't know why it happened any more than I did. But it felt dismissive and planted a seed of shame somewhere inside me.

As my fertility journey unfolded and the first miscarriage proved to be so much more than just a random fluke from a "bad egg," the shame I carried and anger I felt toward my body only compounded.

So, naturally, I set out to fix it. Endless testing and researching later, I made plenty of positive lifestyle changes to reduce inflammation, balance hormones, and support my fertility.

And in many ways, that's a good thing.

However, my relationship with my body started to get kind of wonky as I struggled with fertility. Somewhere along the way, I stopped viewing my body as a gift from God to support and instead saw it as something to fix.

Eventually, the Lord showed me where I was getting it wrong and guided me back to stewarding my body and supporting my fertility from a healthy place and with an appropriate amount of grace.

But I share that honestly because fertility is so closely intertwined with our femininity and our identity. It is a tender and sacred place, and when it is compromised—when it feels like we're unable to do something we are biologically designed to do—it can distort our beliefs about who we are.

If we put our identity in our children (or in our childlessness) more than in our

If we put our identity in our children (or in our childlessness) more than in our being children of God, we run the risk of turning our fertility (and our bodies in general)—a good gift from God to support and steward—into a god.

being children of God, we run the risk of turning our fertility (and our bodies in general)—a good gift from God to support and steward—into a god. As I noted in other chapters, our beliefs and identity deeply influence how we view and treat our bodies. When we are at peace with our bodies, we do not obsess over them or view them as the end themselves. Instead, we can view health and caring for our bodies as a means to an end—to fulfill our callings and bring God glory. But when we resent or obsess over fixing our bodies, they become idols—something to manipulate and control.

Remember, when you're trying to do something entirely on your own, you stop trusting God's sovereignty over all that is out of your control. In my experience, before I know it, my efforts to be healthy or heal something that isn't working right within my body, such as with fertility, can begin to look more like perfectionism and punishment than peaceful stewardship.

FERTILITY FROM A BIBLICAL PERSPECTIVE

Fertility is celebrated and blessed in the Bible. We read in Genesis that the first humans God created were literally told to be fruitful and multiply, yet it seems that nowadays, more women than ever are experiencing reproductive and hormonal problems. According to the WHO, one in six people are affected by infertility.[5] But we're struggling with not just infertility but also other reproductive-related problems like endometriosis, painful periods, and PCOS.

Could this be, at least in part, because our society has gotten so far away from God's original design in areas such food quality, synthetic chemicals, and hormonal birth control pushed on women from a young age (often to remedy a symptom such as irregular cycles)?

Quite possibly. In fact, if we go back to Genesis, we see reproductive challenges are quite literally part of the curse. In Genesis 3:16, God said to the woman, "I will surely multiply your pain in childbearing; in pain you shall bring forth children." For years, I took that literally. I thought it explained why labor and the actual delivery of a baby can be painful. But one day I got curious and decided to dig deeper and I found something profound.

The original Hebrew word for "childbearing" in that verse means not only delivery but also "pregnancy" and "conception."[6] That is, childbearing isn't just the labor and delivery of a child; it's also conception or trying to conceive and pregnancy. According to my research, the original Hebrew word for pain, in this context, is *itzavon,* and it means "'sorrow,' 'grief' and also . . . 'sadness.'"[7]

So if we look at the curse of sin as it relates to women in the context of how the verse was originally written, it is saying that we will have grief, or sorrow, in the whole process of childbearing, not just delivery.

In other words, Genesis 3:16 refers to the agony, hardship, worry, and anxiety of the circumstances in which children are conceived, born, and raised. Old Testament scholar John Walton puts it this way: "Anxiety defines the birth process, even in a world of modern technology and much moreso in the uncertain medical climate of the ancient world. The resulting paraphrase [of Genesis 3:16] would be 'I will greatly increase the anguish you will experience in the birth process, from the anxiety surrounding conception to the strenuous work of giving birth.'"[8]

Wow. *That* changes things. It highlights the reality that no woman escapes this touch of the Fall and curse of sin, though the details for each of us may look different. Some may struggle with pain—grief—when it comes to conception and struggling to conceive. Others may experience it in pregnancy, whether that is by miscarriage, a complication, or a very difficult pregnancy. And still others may experience it in birth or perhaps even after birth, such as through postpartum depression or other conditions.

Motherhood—though it can be very joyful—can also be touched by grief. It is part of the Fall, and that means that because we live between two gardens—Eden and eternity—our motherhood journey here on earth will at some point be affected by brokenness.

When that happens, especially in the circumstances of fertility and pregnancy, are our bodies failing us or our families? No. Our bodies and our families have been failed by sin—by the fall of humanity.

BEING GOOD TO YOUR BODY IS
SUPPORTING YOUR FERTILITY

Some call the menstrual cycle the fifth vital sign, meaning it is a critical health marker. Others refer to fertility as a sign of health in the body. When one or both of these are not working properly, it is safe to assume there is dysfunction happening somewhere internally.

Maybe there's something besides (or in addition to) fertility issues causing you to resent your body. It could be chronic illness, struggles with weight, or anything in between. While working toward healing is a good and worthy thing, don't forget that pursuing health and healing from a broken belief of your body—that it is damaged, unworthy, or a failure—can cause a good intention to spiral into an unhealthy obsession. And there is a very fine line between supporting your body (and fertility) and controlling or even punishing your body for not working properly.

So, where is that line? What is the difference? Let's talk about some practical examples of what supporting your body (and fertility) may look like:

- replenishing minerals and nutrients—in contrast to punishing your body, which may look like restricting calories or major food groups
- prioritizing real, well-sourced food as much as possible—in contrast to punishing your body, which may look like avoiding eating out with friends altogether because the food could be cooked in seed oils or you don't know where it's sourced from
- consuming organic coffee with a balanced breakfast—in contrast to punishing your body, which may look like getting rid of coffee altogether even if it's something you enjoy
- Moving your body in a way you enjoy every day—in contrast to punishing your body, which may look like putting yourself through workouts you genuinely hate

Being good to your body, especially on a fertility journey but even long before or after thinking about pregnancy, *should* include some discipline but *should not* steal your joy. It *should* influence your lifestyle. It *should not* become your whole life.

I could go on, but I'm sure you get the idea.

Supporting your body and your fertility begins with a heart posture of stewardship: "Everything I have—my body, my fertility, my family or future family—is Yours, God." With that truth as the foundation guiding every decision, supporting your body looks like making intentional, God-honoring tweaks to your daily habits, disciplines, and choices to best support where and when you can. But punishing your body is restrictive, manipulative, and controlling. It is often driven by fear and takes all the joy out of the journey. It feels oppressive, like a heavy burden.

Remember, Proverbs 17:22 tells us that "a cheerful heart is good medicine" (NIV). The Bible literally points out that our mental and emotional states can directly influence our health. A cheerful heart—a light spirit not weighed down by burdensome rules and fears—benefits our well-being.

That tells me that being good to your body, especially on a fertility journey but even long before or after thinking about pregnancy, *should* include some discipline but *should not* steal your joy. It *should* influence your lifestyle. It *should not* become your whole life.

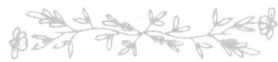

PRAYER

Lord, I ask for guidance in how to best support my body, gently and naturally, regardless of where I am in life or whether it has to do with fertility. Help me to trust You with the timing of my life—to prioritize my health and family over potentially harmful quick fixes. And please give me discernment when it comes to the temporary solutions so readily available for symptoms I may be experiencing, and guard my heart from the allure of hustle and achievement that the world is celebrating. I trust You with my body, my fertility, and my family. Amen.

PRACTICAL APPLICATION

What is one small tweak you can make to your daily disciplines to support your body (and fertility)? Do you have any disciplines or habits that may be too extreme or hard on your body (such as overexercising or undereating)? What about those may need to change to support your well-being in a gentler and more sustainable way?

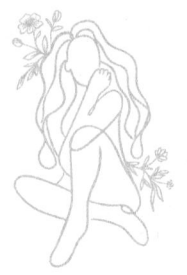

Chapter 12

NOURISH YOUR BODY

I remember throwing a box of hundred-calorie snack packs in my cart during my biweekly grocery run when I was in college. I thought I was being healthy because they were low calorie, and at that time of my life, burning as many and eating as few calories as possible was the goal.

Was I chronically undereating and overexercising? Yes. Did it absolutely wreck my thyroid and hormones? Unfortunately, yes. But I didn't realize that at the time. I just thought I was getting fit and healthy, because, like many of us, I grew up in the nineties and early two thousands when mantras like "A moment on the lips, forever on the hips," low-fat everything, and being skinny were sold as the keys to beauty.

No one talked about minerals and nutrients. Instead of teaching grown women how to meet their body's caloric needs with nutrient-dense meals, culture encouraged us to cut carbs, calories, and anything that could be . . . eek! . . . fattening.

Between the busy culture of today and the diet culture many of us grew up in, I believe that many women have grown accustomed to undereating, even if unintentionally. Of course, many struggle with overeating too. Either way, we've had so much poor messaging and, quite frankly, so many *lies* that influence the way we eat.

The bottom line is that for too long, far too many grown women have primarily thought of health and wellness as restricting calories instead of replenishing nutrients and minerals. We've grown accustomed to eating the bare minimum needed to function and then overindulging because our bodies are crying out to have their needs met. That's when we end up with insane cravings. And in many cases, whether we're undereating or overeating, most of the calories we consume may very well be low in or devoid of nutrients.

Just the other day, I was on Facebook and came across a popular post for a recipe titled Frozen Healthier Snickers. It was a combination of a banana, sugar-free chocolate syrup, caramel syrup, peanut butter, and dry-roasted peanuts. The recipe apparently was *just one point* on WeightWatchers, which a little investigating told me is considered "good." If you're unfamiliar with WeightWatchers, the points system assigns a certain number of points to every food and beverage based on the amounts of calories, sugar, protein, and saturated fats they contain. The lower the points, the "better" the food—which seems to imply that low quantities of the literal fuel our bodies run on, such as calories and saturated fats, are always healthier.

So this sundae is lower points than an actual Snickers bar would be. But is it *healthy*? Instead of labeling a food or product "good" or "bad," let's look at what's in each individual component and see whether it's made of real food ingredients (you know, the stuff

God made and not the processed stuff produced in a lab). Our analysis here isn't based on whether the product is high or low in calories, if it has carbs or not, or any other trendy thing that health culture uses to measure how healthy a food is. Instead, this is the key question: Is it mostly made of what God created, or is it full of man-made, processed, food-*like* ingredients?

When I looked at the chocolate syrup label, I immediately noticed ingredients like artificial flavor and xanthan gum. The caramel syrup was similar. From high-fructose corn syrup to preservatives and artificial food dyes, it was loaded with fillers and additives. Even the peanut butter label included things like dried corn syrup.

Is it mostly made of what God created, or is it full of man-made, processed, food-*like* ingredients?

Aside from the banana, there is very little real food in the recipe. It's packed full of additives, artificial flavors, sweeteners, and dyes. When we actually look at what's in this supposed-to-be-healthy recipe, we can clearly see that there are only trace amounts of real food ingredients. I mean, it is just so far from what God created for our bodies.

So what's the point? The point is that just because something is lower in calories or sugar does not necessarily make it healthy. And that is a prime example of how diet culture and the endless barrage of information online has complicated our understanding of what it means to be good to our bodies.

What's more, it's almost as though half the information we come across is backward. Nutrient-dense food God made, like butter, has been thought of as bad for you because it's more caloric and has saturated fats. But low-calorie food-like products made by humans in a manufacturing plant, such as margarine, have been positioned as "diet friendly" and sold as good for you. It'd be like repeatedly putting the wrong kind of gas in the tank of your car, thinking it's a good thing because of the gas station's good marketing, without realizing it could actually damage the engine.

Let me say this: I'm not claiming to be a nutrition expert, nor am I trying to throw shade on WeightWatchers. Something like WeightWatchers *can* be a helpful starting point for those who truly do need to lose weight to begin their health journey, and the points system can help "gamify" it a bit.

But it doesn't take a nutrition degree to clearly see that recipes like Frozen Healthier Snickers may be low calorie but in no way are truly nourishing, so we need to be careful not to let it be the standard.

All of that said, after looking into the ingredients in this recipe, the question I naturally had was, Why bother to make that kind of thing? I wonder if we'd be better off just eating the Snickers bar instead of going to all the trouble to make a fake one that may be slightly lower in calories but really isn't much healthier. Just eat real, healthy food most of the time and enjoy the treat now and then.

At the very least, it'd be worth saving the time making it and the money buying all the ingredients and would allow us to reinvest those resources into preparing a nutrient-dense *meal* with protein, healthy fat, and quality carbs that actually fuel our bodies.

Another alternative would be to make an actually healthy version with primarily real food ingredients, such as the banana, melted chocolate without all the additives, and an organic peanut butter made with one ingredient: peanuts! No syrups, artificial flavors, or dyes necessary.

There are plenty of other half-truths (or even lies) we've been sold when it comes to what is considered healthy, and that is why we must be diligent and discerning.

REPLENISH INSTEAD OF RESTRICT

What about those of us who want to eat healthily for reasons beyond weight loss, perhaps to help with chronic skin problems or digestive issues?

Not long after my season of chronic undereating and overexercising tendencies, my body began to pay the price of that lifestyle. I uncovered various hormone issues, including a sluggish thyroid and cystic acne.

As I sought to support my thyroid and heal my skin as naturally as possible, there was a period of time when I kind of found myself right back in the habit of intense restriction that more than likely contributed to some of those issues for me in the first place. I tried Whole30 and Paleo. I removed cheese and milk from my diet for years because I'd heard that certain food groups, like dairy, caused acne. For a while, it felt like I was able to eat only a handful of foods because I was low-carb, gluten-free, dairy-free, sugar-free, soy-free, and basically everything-free. And then I began to develop sensitivities to those foods I was eating a lot of, like chickpeas and grapes.

It just felt as if the list of foods that I could eat—even real, God-made foods—kept shrinking. Because I had cut out so many things, I was overloading my body with a small selection of foods, which meant minimal nutrient diversity. In spite of taking multiple supplements to fill in the gaps, mineral testing revealed I was very low in critical nutrients, like calcium.

It wasn't until later that I learned that if I remove something and the problem (like acne) improves, then reintroduce it and the problem comes back, it's possible that all I did was remove a trigger, not heal the true root issue. My dietitian explained it to me like this (at least this is my understanding in non-science layman's terms): Let's say the root cause of a symptom, such as acne, is leaky gut. When I consume a certain food, it seems that I break out more. The natural assumption is that the food is the problem—that it is causing the acne. So it makes sense to remove that food, right? But the leaky gut is still sitting there, unresolved, which means that the true root issue is not healed. While removing triggers may provide some relief or improvement, that is not without downsides, such as the possibility of missing out on highly bio-available nutrients the triggering food group provides.

I had never heard that before! Isn't that so interesting?

Of course, true food allergies are a slightly different conversation, but I was intrigued, and I wondered if perhaps I had only removed triggers without actually solving anything.

I investigated further and learned that, according to Harvard Medical School, glucose is the primary source of energy for cells in our bodies.[1] It's a type of sugar that comes from carbohydrates and proteins that break down during digestion. Glucose is transported into cells with the help of insulin, and it's used by cells along with amino acids and fats to produce energy.[2] So although loading up on refined sugar is obviously not good for our health, restricting all glucose (such as carbs, like some diets suggest) may not be beneficial for our bodies either.

I also learned that the quality and farming practices of certain foods, like dairy products, can make a difference in how they affect our bodies and how we react to them. Without getting into the nitty-gritty details, it's not always the entire food group that is harmful or unhealthy; rather, the culprit might be the way in which it is farmed and sourced.

That was so eye-opening to me because for a long time, I thought that being healthy meant *removing* things—"Avoid sugar; don't eat dairy; carbs and saturated fats are bad!"

But throughout my journey, God showed me that health can actually look like *replenishing*—adding more good things to my plate. And as good things—nutrient-dense, God-made fuel—began to fill my plate, there was less room (and even less desire or craving) for the not-so-good things.

Here's what I mean by that: When I'm eating nutrient-dense calories and meeting my daily protein needs, hydrating, and supporting my sleep, I feel better and find that I don't reach for food loaded with fillers and devoid of nutrients.

When I shifted my approach, things changed. Instead of restricting calories or foods that diet culture labeled as bad (like butter, sugar, and carbs), I just tried to replenish my body with more whole, God-made foods. The only "foods" I tried to minimize were the ones that were not actually food—the items that were edible but not beneficial, such as food-like products loaded with artificial colors, flavors, and preservatives. Unsurprisingly, that happens to be when my skin began to clear, my hormones balanced out, and my natural energy improved.

> God showed me that health can actually look like *replenishing*—adding more good things to my plate. And as good things—nutrient-dense, God made fuel—began to fill my plate, there was less room (and even less desire or craving) for the not-so-good things.

BEING GOOD TO YOUR BODY IS GIVING IT THE FUEL IT NEEDS

I drive a 2014 Jeep Grand Cherokee. Yep, it's more than ten years old. It's nothing fancy. It has 150,000 miles on it and a few dings and scratches in the paint. There are little snack puffs and various other odds and ends (from my kids) lodged deep between the seats. I have had several opportunities to upgrade, but I just haven't been eager to do so. I mean, sure, my car isn't the latest or the greatest, but it runs well and I've done my best to take care of it. I take it in for regular oil changes (well, my husband does, but you know what I mean), fill the gas tank with the right kind of fuel, try to keep it clean-ish, and make sure to have routine maintenance done on it.

It won't last me forever. It will eventually take its last drive. But she (yes, I decided it's a girl Jeep—don't judge me) has been good to me because I've been good to her.

Not to make another car metaphor, but my body isn't all that different from that Jeep. If I give my body the fuel, or food, that it needs, it will be able to run well. But if I expect it to essentially run on fumes (like caffeine and cortisol) by my living in a chronic state of stress, breakdown is going to happen.

What do I mean by running on fumes?

I turned to my dietitian and friend, Robyn, for an answer. Here's how she explained it:

When the primary source of energy for our bodies is nutrient-dense food, the body uses that as fuel. Food is the body's preferred source of energy—especially protein, fat, and carbs. But the body has backup mechanisms for energy, such as cortisol. If the body is under stress for extended periods of time, which can be caused by things like undereating (or restricting calories), poor sleep, overworking, or overexercising, the body can default to these backup mechanisms, instead of food, for energy. That can negatively impact our metabolism, which can negatively impact our weight and energy.

So, running on fumes essentially means running on stress hormones instead of fuel from food. Too bad they don't let me put emojis in books, because this is where I would type the little "mind blown" guy.

I mean, wow. Many of us are just used to living in a state of chronic stress. Often, we don't even realize it. And instead of running on nutrient-dense food, rich in vitamins and minerals, our bodies begin to run on fumes—on those backup mechanisms Robyn mentioned. *Stress hormones.*

Consider stewardship, which begins with palms up, hands open, and heart in a posture that says, "Everything I have is Yours, God."

If I believe that every resource I have, including my body (or, in this metaphor, my car), belongs to the Lord, how much more likely am I to give it the fuel *He* created and provided for it? If He provides the car and the fuel (the gift of a good body and good fuel it needs to function optimally), it only makes sense to give our bodies the proper fuel they need.

Scripture lays out very clearly the food God gave us as fuel. In Genesis 1:29, He said, "Behold, I have given you every plant yielding seed that is on the face of all the earth, and every tree with seed in its fruit. You shall have them for food." And in Genesis 9:3, He said, "Every moving thing that lives shall be food for you. And as I gave you the green plants, I give you everything."

Translation: The foods God gave for our bodies as fuel are fruits, root vegetables, various greens, grains, and animal protein.

Our world may try to replicate or make various fake versions of those things. Or it may take what God created and genetically modify it, add preservatives, or add artificial additives—such as flavoring or dyes or other unnecessary additions to make a good thing more addictive, convenient, or shelf-stable—sometimes to the point that what began as a real food is no longer recognizable.

While no food is perfect, as we live in a fallen world—and as a result it can be very difficult to completely avoid all food that has been affected by the fallen nature of our world—the best we can do is our best. We can do our due diligence and be thoughtful about the way we support our bodies' natural energy and give them the fuel they need.

Are we running on fumes or severely restricting calories and whole food groups that are God-given sources of fuel, such as nourishing carbs (for example, fruit and potatoes)? Or are we replenishing and fueling our bodies with the appropriate amount of food and type of nutrients they need?

That doesn't mean never again eating boxed mac and cheese or pizza or whatever else may not be made of good, whole, unadulterated ingredients. But it *does* mean that it's our job to do what we can to prioritize nourishing our bodies with proper fuel. And how much you are able to do may look different from what your friend or neighbor does, and that's okay.

PRAYER

God, it can be so easy to get tangled up in all the fad diets and health trends in society. I have been guilty of listening to the world more than I lean into Your Word. But I trust that the food You made is the most nourishing for my body. You designed all of creation—including my body—perfectly, and I know that my responsibility is to give my body the fuel You created for it. Thank You for the food You provide for me. I know that this world is fallen and all food is touched by the Fall in some way, but please help me be willing to go out of my way to find the best quality and nourish my body with the real food You made for it to eat. From this point on, I commit to nourishing my body appropriately with the proper fuel instead of running on stress hormones, or fumes. I will do my best not to skip meals because I'm too busy or overeat junk that doesn't fuel my body well. Amen.

PRACTICAL APPLICATION

Find one way to incorporate more nutrient-dense foods into your diet. Maybe start with incorporating nourishing snacks in place of heavily processed ones. For example, instead of eating popcorn or chips before bed, consider some protein, carbs, and healthy fat. I personally love to have orange slices or berries with some cottage cheese or Greek yogurt for a bit of protein. Or maybe instead of a bowl of cereal for breakfast, could you have some eggs, yogurt, and avocado slices or fruit? Whatever you choose, start with one shift in your daily habits to incorporate more nourishment.

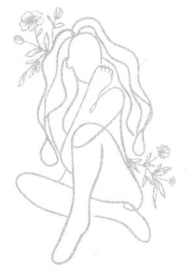

Chapter 13

MOVE YOUR BOOTY

For most of my life, I've had a complicated relationship with fitness. The more conversations I have with friends and other thirty-plus women, the more I realize how many of us have been in the same boat. Yet we hardly talk about this part of wellness.

I feel like we hear and talk a lot about complicated relationships with our bodies or with food, which is absolutely an important part of the conversation, but we don't talk much about the exercise component. So I want to chat about it because many of us have struggled or are currently struggling with finding the right routine and balance without leaning too far into either inactivity *or* over-exercising.

If you're anything like me, you may have flip-flopped between one and the other.

As I shared early on in this book, there were several years of my life (especially in my early twenties) that I was obsessed with working out. I exercised constantly—tracked every calorie I burned and every step I took, thanks to my Apple Watch. I ran long distances every day, spent hours upon hours in the gym, and would not allow myself to skip a workout even if that meant working out at 11:00 P.M. if that was the only "free" time I had in a day. Have you ever gone through a phase like that?

Week after week, I became more and more lean. I posted photos of my flexed abs on my social media pages to show my progress (which have since been deleted and shall never see the light of day ever again).

I came to understand that exercise *can* be a stressor on the body, especially too much exercise when the body is already in a stressed-out state (undernourished, sleep deprived, and so on).

Fitness was my god. And for the most part, it stayed that way until I struggled to have a baby. As I researched and learned more about my body's biological needs, specifically regarding fitness, I came to understand that exercise *can* be a stressor on the body, especially too much exercise when the body is already in a stressed-out state (undernourished, sleep deprived, and so on). That was fascinating to me because I'd only ever thought of exercise as a way to *reduce* stress. Never once had I considered that daily high-intensity interval training (HIIT) could possibly be *adding* stress to my system.

When my testing revealed that I had adrenal fatigue and hormone imbalance, I began to slow down on my fitness routine a bit. Fast-forward a couple of years and I finally got pregnant with my son, the first baby I carried to term. However, I was put on blood thinners and a pretty strict protocol due to my pregnancy-loss history, which meant I was not supposed to work out or even lift more than a gallon of milk for the first fourteen weeks.

I (a generally very active person) had to be almost completely sedentary for the first time in as long as I could remember. Although I looked forward to getting a little more active again when I passed the fourteen-week mark, I was terrified to "mess anything up" after a history of so much loss, so I didn't push it. I was exhausted and it was also the middle of winter, so I ended up staying pretty inactive for the remainder of my pregnancy.

Then, I thought for sure I would get back into working out as soon as I was cleared six weeks postpartum. But my birth plan went sideways and I ended up having a C-section and a very fussy baby who basically never slept. Additionally, we had just recently adopted my (slightly) older son, so we were raising two babies under one year old and I breastfed both of them. So when I was six weeks postpartum, working out was the last thing my tired and still-recovering body had any energy for.

A few more weeks went by. Then a few months. Before I knew it, I found myself nearly one year postpartum, still not very active and not at all motivated to exercise anymore. It got to a point where I pretty much felt nervous to try to get back into any kind of routine. It may sound silly, but it was like I was afraid to see how far I had regressed—how out of shape I was after more than eighteen months of inactivity (outside of taking care of babies).

I had nothing to prove to anyone. No one was standing there judging me if I couldn't jog a mile without stopping or wasn't able to do as many repetitions as I used to be able to. But I was judging myself.

It sounds so ridiculous, but my fear of embarrassing myself in front of . . . myself? . . . held me back from returning to a workout routine that I desperately missed and needed. Plus, with my history of overexercising and obsession with fitness and my tendency to want to do all or nothing, a small part of me was unsure how to get back into exercise without overdoing it.

But then a friend gently reminded me that it doesn't need to be all or nothing, and one Tuesday afternoon, something came over me and I found the courage to begin again.

Slowly, with a small step.

My very first workout after a long time off was a walk-jog around my neighborhood. I would walk a hundred yards, then jog a hundred yards, so on and so forth for one mile.

I was winded the whole time, and the next day I was sore. That was hard for me—a shot to my pride—because a walk-jog like that used to be my warm-up just a couple of years prior.

I knew I had a long way to go, but as humbling as that first workout was, I felt all the more determined to get some of my strength and endurance back.

MAKING A MOVEMENT PLAN

I put together a plan I felt I could stick to: two or three light but intentional workouts a week. I worked in more strength training than I ever had before, instead of just focusing on cardio. And as I did, I was reminded of a woman I used to see every day at the gym I went to years before I had babies. She was so strong. So fit. She did some impressive workouts at six o'clock each morning. And I was intimidated by her—until I actually talked to her one day. She told me that she had committed herself to getting her strength back after multiple C-sections. At the time, I respected that but truly didn't understand what she meant or what that was like.

Now I deeply understood exactly what she meant and why it was so important to her to feel strong again. After having a C-section and experiencing how difficult the recovery was and re-alizing how much strength I truly lost, I felt that same desire and determination she did.

Naturally, I wanted to commit to regaining *my* strength, too, in a way that would be sustainable and with some bumpers to prevent obsession, given my history with working out.

Some of those built-in boundaries looked like this:

- I committed to no less than two workouts per week and no more than five.
- I worked out with a buddy as much as possible for accountability.
- I set clear and measurable strength (not weight or pants-size) goals, such as being able to do five push-ups.
- I exercised in a way that was appropriate for where I was at in my menstrual cycle (some call this "cycle syncing"). For example, I focused on gentler movement (like incline walking and strength training) during my luteal and menstrual phase and incorporated more cardio (like full-body conditioning and jogging) during my follicular and ovulation phases.

Guidelines like that helped me stay consistent and stick to my commitment without falling into my old patterns of obsession and overexercising. I signed up for Burn Boot Camp and began to go twice a week with my sister-in-law. In between classes and before my kids wake up or during their naps, I do light workouts at home, such as incline walking on the treadmill. I take at least two days off each week to focus on rest and recovery.

At the time of writing this, it's been a few months of this new routine. Six months ago, I could hardly do a push-up. Today, I can do more than five at one time without having to switch to my knees! Huzzah! After years of miscarriages and grief, an endometriosis diagnosis, a high-risk pregnancy, a C-section recovery, raising two babies, and a long period of inactivity, that's a win for me. I feel energized. I'm getting my strength back. I don't feel weak or fatigued when I lift my twenty-five-pound toddlers anymore.

And that's what I'm doing it all for anyway—increasing my strength and stamina is an investment into my energy and ability to care for my family—to fulfill my calling.

I *feel* like myself again for the first time in a long time, but a healthier, nourished, more deeply rooted version of me, where Jesus, not fitness, is on the throne. Fitness used to be a tool for making my body look a certain way. Now? It's simply one of many methods for supporting my body and overall well-being.

Not to look flawless but to *live fully*.

Not for vanity but for *vitality*.

Not to be skinny but to be *strong*.

Not for looking extra lean but for my *family*.

Like any good thing, fitness can be abused. I know from personal experience that it's possible to overdo it. But the truth is that movement is a gift. The ability to exercise is a privilege that shouldn't be taken lightly. And just because it *can* be taken too far or be a stressor on the body if not done in such a way that works with our female physiology doesn't mean it should be avoided entirely. Exercise is an integral, undeniable part of being good to our bodies.

> Movement is an integral, undeniable part of being good to our bodies.

BEING GOOD TO YOUR BODY IS MOVING

The Bible is very clear about the importance of movement and physical training. As we've already discussed, we know that Genesis tells us that man was set in a garden and instructed to keep it and tend to it (see 2:15). I bring that up again here because tending to a garden is a physical task.

While they didn't have Planet Fitness or Burn Boot Camp classes in biblical times, it's evident from that verse alone that we were made to move—to work with our hands and be physically active.

Nowadays, that often looks like going to the gym or setting aside time for a formal workout. Many of us spend a significant amount of time sitting, whether driving or working at a desk, but we were designed for a lifestyle of movement.

Moreover, various other places in Scripture emphasize the importance of moving our bodies. As I've mentioned before, Proverbs 31:17 tells us that a virtuous woman "dresses herself with strength and makes her arms strong." Strength can be both spiritual and physical, and I personally believe that description speaks to both.

I also think of 1 Timothy 4:8: "While bodily training is of some value, godliness is of value in every way, as it holds promise for the present life and also for the life to come." That reminds me that physical training matters and is valuable, but not to the extent that we sacrifice the fruit of the Spirit—"love, joy, peace, patience, kindness, goodness, faithfulness, gentleness, self-control" (Galatians 5:22–23)—for it. While physical fitness is important, it is not ultimate.

If it becomes an obsession that steals our joy or peace, it may be time to make a shift. Our movement should be a response to our creator and flow from the fruit of the Spirit. Maybe it's my competitive nature, but I spent way too long believing the lie that fitness had to be a competition—like beating my last time or personal record or being the fastest or the strongest in the class, whether it was spin, Pilates, or something else. Slowly, I began to let go of that need to "win" or "beat" anyone (including myself) and instead started to move my body from a place of worship and obedience.

Don't get me wrong, a little healthy competition can be motivating sometimes. But it can also lead to obsession and distract us from the whole point of exercise. In fact, if we feel there is a competition we can't win—even if it's a competition we made up in our heads that no one else in the gym or class is aware of—we are much more likely to sit out. In the process, our egos rob our bodies of their need for exercise, like mine did when I was resistant to getting back into a routine after having a baby.

However, if we learn to view exercise as an act of obedience, as a crucial part of stewardship, it will become a healthy rhythm in holistically godly lives without turning into the god of our lives.

> If we learn to view exercise as an act of obedience, as a crucial part of stewardship, it will become a healthy rhythm in holistically godly lives without turning into the god of our lives.

Want to be good to your body? Consider creating a *realistic* exercise plan that you can stick to, even if it's only one or two times a week to begin. Ask for help. Team up with a friend for some accountability.

But however you can and whatever you do, *move*.

And in every breath and every bead of sweat, give God glory and practice gratitude for the gift of your good body.

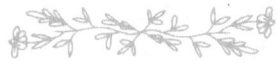

PRAYER

God, I know that I am made to move, and I want to be disciplined and consistent when it comes to exercise. Help me not rely on motivation or stumble into obsession but rather move my body in worship of and response to You. I am grateful for the gift of my body, and I know that choosing to move my body however I can is a way to live out that gratitude. I pray for discernment and discipline in this area and ask You to guide me as I seek to establish sustainable and healthy routines for moving my body. Amen.

PRACTICAL APPLICATION

If you don't currently have a workout routine, create a realistic one you can stick with, even if you start with just two days a week.

If you already have a routine, take a moment to consider if it is more supportive or more stressful to your body. Is it mainly high-intensity cardio workouts? Are you allowing yourself regular recovery and rest days? Do you feel peace when you take a day off, or does it bother you? If your workout is more stressful than supportive, what modifications might you be able to implement in order to make it as supportive as possible to your hormones and feminine physiology?

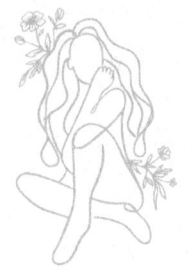

Chapter 14

KNOW YOUR NEIGHBORS

I walked into a local café today to work on this chapter. It's one of my favorite spots and I've spent an embarrassing amount of time here over the past several months whenever I can sneak away from home to work.

"Hi, Jordan!" the barista called as I walked through the door. "How are the boys?"

I said hi, filled him in on the kids' latest milestones, and chatted with him for a bit about various things before I placed my order.

Then, a few minutes later, the owner herself brought me my drink. I had purchased a few decor items from the shop in the front of the café a few weeks prior for my younger son's birthday party, so she asked how the celebrations went.

After she walked away, as I was sipping on my iced matcha latte, it struck me: It's such a gift to be noticed, known, and cared about in my local community!

THE IMPORTANCE OF COMMUNITY

When you think of healthy living, what comes to mind? Nutritious food? Filtered water? A workout routine? Quality sleep?

Those are all important things. But there is an often overlooked yet vital *good thing* that our bodies and hearts need: relationship. If you're anything like me, that may feel like the hardest one to achieve. Drinking enough water, choosing a nutrient-dense meal, and going to bed earlier are things I can control for myself. But building community? It requires someone else's response. It's a two-way street, doesn't always come easy, and can feel intimidating.

For years, friendships felt so fickle for me. It seemed like I would be close with someone one minute and then life circumstances would change and she'd be spending most of her time with a new guy or new friend group. Or one of us would move or enter into a new season, and the friendship would shift or fade.

Maybe you know the feeling.

I desired meaningful relationships and a supportive community, and I slowly worked to cultivate those relationships throughout my twenties. Some friendships were constant, others came and went, and still others didn't last beyond a short season.

But then, on my thirtieth birthday, a couple of my friends gathered all the local women I love to celebrate with me at a local winery on a beautiful summer evening. And as we listened to live music while enjoying charcuterie and birthday cake (*without* stressing about ingredients or calories), I looked around the table of familiar faces, many of whom walked with me through years of grief, and realized I had the community I once prayed for.

Although friends like these have been an answered prayer and huge blessing, I have also learned that building community doesn't look only like a group of like-minded women. That's one type of community, and an important one at that. Although it's worth patiently investing in, building community doesn't always happen quickly and can be hard to create, especially in seasons of a demanding school or work schedule or raising families and having little time to dedicate to visiting.

So, how else can we cultivate a village—a sense of community and belonging?

In addition to strengthening multigenerational relationships within our own families (when possible), some of my favorite ways to connect with a community include shopping or dining at locally owned businesses, plugging into a church, getting to know my neighbors (even if they don't become my closest friends), and sourcing food from local farms.

SHOP SMALL, SUPPORT LOCAL

My husband is a foodie in every sense of the word, and he enjoys getting to know the owners of local coffee shops, cafés, and restaurants because, as he says, "I love seeing people care so much about their craft, whether it's perfecting latte art or making the best pork chop in town."

As we find our favorite spots, we return to them regularly and, as a result, establish relationships with the owners, staff, and other regulars. Now when we walk into our favorite coffee shop, we're not only greeted as a guest but also known by name. As the baristas take our order, they ask about the kids, how a project we've been working on is going, or about other parts of our lives that we've shared. Are they our best friends? Do we hang out with them on Friday nights? No, but we do feel *known*. And that meets a basic human need: to be known and seen. And believe it or not, supporting local businesses and becoming a "regular" is a way to create that connection and the sense of belonging we all crave. And sometimes it leads to connections that turn into friendships beyond the walls of the restaurant or coffee shop.

Similarly, as we regularly attend and get involved in a local church, connections are naturally made. Maybe not in the first weeks, but slowly, as we show up consistently, relationships begin to unfold. My husband and I personally chose a smallish church and intentionally reached out to the leadership there early on to get plugged in and connected instead of passively attending. Then, as we gradually began to recognize familiar faces and be recognized in return, we were able to organically build friendships that grew beyond Sunday service and outside the church walls.

Additionally, we enjoy going to the farmers' market not only because we can buy local organic produce but also because it's a fun family activity and connects us to our community. We run into neighbors and catch up with people from church, discover new small businesses, and support and buy from local farmers to source higher-quality eggs, dairy, meat, and produce than we could find at the grocery store.

Those are just a few examples that work for me. However you choose to find community, know that biblically and scientifically, it is a critical part of health and well-being.

THE SCIENCE BEHIND COMMUNITY AND THE BODY

As my journey to wellness unfolded, I found that being good to my body was more than tossing out products with toxic ingredients or eating organic. Equally important are relationships, plugging into my community, and sourcing locally.

Did you know that evidence links perceived loneliness and social isolation with depression, poor sleep quality, and impaired executive function?[1] In other words, isolation can have a negative impact on our mental and emotional well-being, and that can affect us physically.

On the other hand, getting more involved in our local communities and having healthy social relationships can benefit our health greatly. I mean, have you heard of the Roseto effect?

The Roseto effect is a phenomenon that describes how close-knit communities may experience lower rates of heart disease. The effect was first noticed in 1961 by researchers who observed that the Italian American community of Roseto, Pennsylvania, had an unusually low rate of myocardial infarction compared to other areas. Further research, including blood-sample testing, found that people in Roseto had a 50 percent higher chance of survival than those with weaker social ties and that men over age sixty-five in Roseto had a heart disease death rate that was roughly half the national average. Researchers also found that there was no leading cause of death in Roseto and that people were dying of old age.[2]

Moreover, according to the Mayo Clinic, meaningful relationships provide numerous benefits, like reducing stress, helping us cope with hard times, and providing support and accountability to help one another change or avoid unhealthy lifestyle habits, such as excessive drinking or lack of exercise. "Adults with strong social connections have a lower risk of many health problems. That includes depression, high blood pressure and an unhealthy weight. In fact, studies have found that older adults who have close friends and healthy social supports are likely to live longer than do their peers who have fewer friends."[3]

Not only have I learned that social relationships benefit one's sense of joy, belonging, and decision-making, but I've also found that plugging into our local community, such as through farmers' markets, can lead to healthier choices for sourcing groceries and homemade staples. The bottom line is that various research and studies confirm that investing time and energy into building meaningful relationships and getting plugged into a local community bring various benefits when it comes to health and well-being.

The Bible confirms connection and community as basic human needs. God Himself said that it's not good for man to be alone, so He did something about that by creating Eve. He made *woman* to be the catalyst for community.

> Investing time and energy into building meaningful relationships and getting plugged into our local community bring various benefits when it comes to health and well-being.

The need for relationship and connection is at the foundation of our creation; it is part of the purpose for which we were created. It should be no surprise that feminine physiology is nurturing and relational by nature.

You know what that means for you and me? We could do all the things we've discussed so far about living a healthy life—like eating right, moving our bodies, hydrating—and still be miserable and less than healthy if we are isolated and lonely.

Being part of a community is key to being good to our bodies because it is one of the *good things* that God created in the beginning of human history to meet one of our most basic needs.

Having relationships also encourages slower living in a fast-paced society where we have grown to rely on conveniences, rush to and from work, and rarely stop to talk to our neighbors. (Unless you're from the Midwest; Midwesterners are infamous for being genuinely nice. My husband, an Arizona native, claims that must be because our ancestors needed one another to survive the winters. Ha!)

So if you want to be good to your body, invest in your local community. You may not find all your best friends overnight, but get to know your neighbors. Bake them some brownies or take over a casserole. Support your local farmer. Strike up a conversation with a local coffee shop owner. One connection at a time can lead to another, and over time, you may find that you have a village surrounding you.

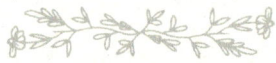

PRAYER

God, I believe I am made in Your image and that You are relational by nature. I want to do a better job of going out of my way to get plugged into my local community, know my neighbors, and source resources from small businesses and farms near me. I ask for wisdom and discernment as I seek out local businesses and farms I might consider supporting and as I intentionally try to make connections with people around me. Give me the courage to introduce myself, get out of my comfort zone, and engage in the community that surrounds me. I pray for meaningful friendships with like-minded people who support me, love me, sharpen me, and make me more like You, and I pray that I can be that for them too. Help me be patient and trust that You are working, even if a tight-knit community does not form overnight. I trust You to lead the way, and I ask You to guide me as I intentionally look for ways to plug into my community day after day. Amen.

PRACTICAL APPLICATION

- *Find your local farmers' market and start doing some of your grocery shopping there each week. You can find farmers' markets near you by going to www .localfarmmarkets.org.*
- *Sign up for a book club or workout class that sounds interesting. You don't need to make a new best friend right off the bat. Just meet some people and get to know them during the weekly meetings or classes.*
- *Make a meal for your neighbors and take it over to them or invite them over for a meal (even if you've never talked to them before!).*
- *Become a "regular" at a local business you like, whether that's a coffee shop, restaurant, hair salon, boutique, or something else. Intentionally take the time to set your phone down and engage with those who work there.*

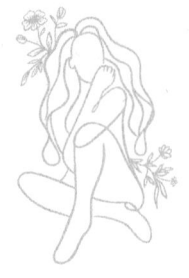

Chapter 15

INVEST IN YOUR HEALTH

There's something we need to talk about: the *financial* side of being good to your body.

Ideally, creating a healthy lifestyle would be free and easy—natural, really. And at one time it was. Adam and Eve didn't have to go to the same lengths to care for their bodies before the Fall as we do now. Creation was unadulterated, void of pesticides and Big Pharma and money and the food industry and all the other things that can have negative health implications in our world today.

Adam and Eve just lived in perfect peace, all their food was nourishing, and everything they needed was provided—freely given. I look forward to the day when God restores all things and our bodies are redeemed—when it will be that way again. But as we live "in between" in this fallen world, we face all sorts of things in our daily lives that can take a toll on our well-being.

Are there changes we can make and things we can do to reduce and improve those things? Totally. As we've discussed, we can buy air purifiers, shop for products with safer ingredients on the labels, filter our water, source organic, shop locally, and so on and so forth.

But are those things free? No, far from it. In fact, sometimes they're not even very affordable. In some places, they're difficult to find. The hard and sad reality is that in today's world, we have gotten so far from God's original design for our bodies to thrive that it can actually be more costly to live a little more naturally than conventionally—or so it seems.

Cultivating healthy environments, fueling our bodies with real food, and sourcing products with safer ingredients isn't cheap. It's less convenient, which means it takes more of our time too.

That poses a real challenge for us, especially in the conversation regarding stewardship. What are we supposed to do if we want to make changes and live more healthfully (to be good stewards of our *bodies*) but also want to ensure we live within our means (to be good stewards of our *money*)? It's tricky!

Is spending money on your health a worthy investment? Absolutely. However, if it gets to a point where you're driving yourself or your family into a financial crisis in the process, the stress that may accompany that could have just as much of a negative impact on your health as genetically modified organisms (GMOs) and toxins.

So what do we do about it? Let money dictate the decisions we make for our bodies? That doesn't sound like a great option. But what about if the alternative is that the pursuit of health or healing leads us to financial stress? That sounds like an equally bad option.

As a reminder, stewardship entails viewing all we have—our bodies, our families, our health, our resources, our money—as God's and treating it accordingly.

That means that being good to our bodies includes being wise with our money, which really belongs to God and is entrusted to us to manage. Our bodies and our money are not mutually exclusive. You cannot steward one and neglect the other. They must work together.

WHY IS HEALTHY STUFF SO EXPENSIVE?

We often ask why safer products are so expensive. But what if the question we should be asking is, Why are unsafe products so *cheap*?

I read a *Vogue* article about why things like clean beauty products are generally more expensive than their conventional counterparts. I mean, you would assume that if a product is more natural, if it comes from nature, it should be cheaper, right? You can just go out and find a virtually unlimited amount of ingredients from the earth, right? Not exactly.

For example, "there can be a much longer research and development timeline involved, especially if a brand is trying to create a clean version of an existing product. This can contribute to a higher overall price point." Additionally, in conventional products, active ingredients are often preserved with things like parabens and propylene glycol. Those are not considered safe, and therefore safer product lines have to utilize different raw materials and preservation methods, which can lead to higher costs to produce and therefore a higher price for the end consumer.

Then, toward the end of the article, one of the interviewees, Siddharth Somaiya, says, "We have gotten used to buying junk, which is why there is a misconception that clean beauty is expensive in comparison. . . . It is important to remember that when you're buying safe skincare, we are buying from people who are foregoing a lot of profitability in order to provide quality products, in terms of harvesting and extraction methods."[1]

Did you catch that? *We have gotten used to buying junk,* which is why there is a misconception that cleaner products are expensive by comparison.

INVESTMENT > EXPENSE

Have you ever read the parable of the talents in the Bible? In a nutshell, a wealthy master gives his assets to three servants and tells them to invest them while he's away on a long trip. When he returns, he rewards the servants based on how they used their resources. Two servants, referred to as the faithful servants, double the value of their investments and are rewarded with, "Well done, good and faithful servant. You have been faithful over a little; I will set you over much" (Matthew 25:21). But one servant buries the money out of fear and does nothing with it. As a result, he does not earn a return. The master condemns him as "wicked and slothful" (verse 26) and casts him out.

What can we learn from that? What's the meaning of the story? The message is that Jesus's servants should wisely invest the resources given to them.

Additionally, we see in Proverbs 31:16 that the virtuous woman "considers a field and buys it." Rather than being hasty with her money or purchasing something frivolously, she gives careful thought to the transaction. After buying the field, she uses it for a productive purpose.

How does that apply to us when it comes to spending money, especially on our health? Does it literally mean that every expenditure needs to lead to financial profits or doubling that money to be God honoring? Of course not. But I would argue that there is wisdom in investing in things that yield a reward or bring forth valuable fruit, whether that fruit is financial, relational, spiritual, or physical. Rather than hoarding money because of fear, there is biblical wisdom in investing in the things that will improve and bring value to our lives and the lives of others.

Perhaps a differentiator between a frivolous expense and a wise investment is whether it leads to fruit. Is there a productive purpose? Does it lead to long-term gain or benefit? If so, it's more likely wise than frivolous.

> Rather than hoarding money because of fear, there is biblical wisdom in investing in the things that will improve and bring value to our lives and the lives of others.

We often think of investing in terms of just actual dollars and cents. If I invest in a real estate property, hold on to it, and sell it for a profit ten years later, that's a good investment, right?

If a piece of land that yields a generous reward is considered a worthy investment, how much worthier is the investment of resources (even money) in the vessels in which we carry out our God-given callings—our bodies? Perhaps we need to reframe the way we view spending money on our well-being. Instead of seeing it as an expense, or a sunk cost, let's instead understand and treat it as an investment. Spending money on your or your family's health is not a frivolous cost or expense like a shopping spree might be. It's an investment into your current and long-term well-being, which, according to Scripture, is evidence of virtue and faithfulness. Investing wisely is a good thing.

In fact, some would argue that we'll pay either way—either up front, by investing in better-quality or safer products, or on the back end, in medical bills from treatments for health issues. I understand the sentiment, and in many cases it's probably accurate. However, we have to acknowledge that there are plenty of people who make the investment in their health in every way possible and still get sick or face health challenges. I fear we may be setting ourselves up for disappointment if we tell ourselves that if we just bite the bullet and spend the money from the get-go, we'll be able to avoid any and all problems and illness. No one gets out of this life unscathed—or alive, for that matter. However, are those who actively invest in their health and well-being *less* likely to face health issues, statistically? Yes.

With that in mind, being a good steward of both our bodies and our money go hand in hand. And at the end of the day, using resources like money for the purpose of supporting our present and future health and improving our well-being is far from a frivolous expense; it is an *investment*.

EXPENSIVE OR INCONVENIENT?

When I began to make various lifestyle changes to be better to my body, from shopping for safer products to sourcing more food locally, it seemed so costly. So much more expensive. And although there were absolutely things that did cost more monetarily, I began to realize that it was indeed possible to make some changes on a budget. But it wasn't necessarily easy, because it was not very *convenient*. In many cases, I had to go out of my way or take some time out of my day to pick up local pasture-raised eggs or grass-fed milk.

When I broke down the dollars and cents of it, the cost of grabbing those things at the store (or, let's be real, having them delivered via Instacart) and joining a local Community Supported Agriculture (CSA) program or herd share (where people buy shares of a milking animal or herd and pay the farmer to care for the animals and milk them) were actually quite comparable. Yes, if I were to buy the top-of-the-line, pasture-raised eggs available at the grocery store, that would have cost more than if I'd grabbed the conventional eggs on the shelf right next to them. However, if I sourced them from a small local farm, it actually didn't cost much more. (Note: I had previously done my homework to research which local farm to patronize.) In fact, there were some cases where something like a carton of eggs cost less by sourcing this way.

I think we automatically assume that healthier options are always more expensive. If you compare the conventional produce and organic produce sitting next to each other on a grocery store shelf, the organic is always going to cost more, yet that doesn't mean there aren't ways to find these healthier alternatives at a more affordable price.

As I learned, sometimes doing things a little differently to source quality food or other products is not necessarily always more expensive but can be inconvenient (or, at least, *less* convenient).

It takes some research to find farms to source from. It also requires integrating local farm pickups into your schedule or going to the farmers' market when it's open. It can require us to go out of our way to seek out the best quality that we can find while staying within our means. I know, it sounds a little extra, but as I've already mentioned, if we look at the Bible, isn't that what the Proverbs 31 woman did? As a reminder, verse 14 (which we briefly talked about in chapter 3) says, "She is like the ships of the merchant; she brings her food from afar."

While thoughts on the specific interpretations of this verse vary among scholars, I did a little digging on my own and a few consistent themes emerged when looking at commentaries:

- The Proverbs 31 woman doesn't settle for what's convenient.
- She will go out of her way to provide the best food for her family.
- She travels far to find bargains or, at minimum, the best price.
- She searches widely for what she buys.

Obviously, there are only so many hours in a day, and grocery delivery can be a beautiful gift. No shame in taking advantage of it if it makes sense for you financially. However, when we're considering stewardship of both the physical body and our finances, the Proverbs 31 woman has a lot to teach those of us who live in a world of Instacart and same-day shipping.

From other context clues in the passage, we can conclude that she is wise with her money, so it can't be implied that she just buys the best of everything regardless of what it does to her family financially. But she is *thoughtful* about what she spends her resources on and doesn't just choose the easiest thing if there are better options.

The world is obsessed with convenience and may even poke fun at a woman for being high-maintenance if she looks for regenerative farming practices, cooks from scratch, or is choosy about the products she spends her money on or brings into her home. So Proverbs 31 is just a reminder that, biblically, inconvenience does not equal bad and having high standards does not necessarily make someone high-maintenance. Can our search for the best quality get out of hand or turn into an unhealthy obsession? Of course. As we've already discussed, anything can. But just because that's a possibility does not mean we should throw all standards or thoughtfulness about these things out the window.

It *does* matter how we spend our resources and feed our families. The details of what each of us will be able to do will vary based on our unique situations, seasons of life, and budgets. That's a given. But the Bible is clear that being thoughtful and seeking the best quality is godly.

Having high standards does not necessarily make someone high-maintenance.

And we, as women who are the wives and mothers of our families, have an important, God-appointed role to be the gatekeepers of our home. Being the gatekeepers of our homes requires using wisdom to decide who and what gets to contribute to our families' values, meaning what comes into our homes through TV shows, social media, relationships, and the products we use and foods we consume. All those things affect our mental, emotional, and physical well-being.

So, is being thoughtful about our wellness bougie? Is it just being super crunchy? Too picky?

Or is it actually biblical, part of a high and holy calling?

I'd argue that with a healthy heart posture, it's the latter.

That doesn't mean we can control everything, should live beyond our means, or must buy all the top-shelf, highest-quality products if that doesn't make sense financially. It *does* mean that it is our duty to be wise and, when possible, go the extra mile for our well-being and that of our families instead of always settling for what's quick, convenient, cheap, and easy.

The following question might step on some toes, but I'm going to ask it in love: Is it possible that we avoid the inconvenience of looking for better options where we can because we've made up our minds ahead of time that it's just going to be too expensive? Is it an excuse we tell ourselves to avoid the work it can take to find better options that would fit into our budget? Do we believe the lie that if we can't afford it all, if we can't change everything, we might as well change nothing? I know I've been guilty of that before.

Rather than automatically avoiding possibly healthier alternatives out of fear that something is out of our means, it is far better to look at our finances, do some digging, and find where we can afford to make some healthy changes, even if it's doing just one or two things differently at first.

I get that much of what you'd like to do might not be realistic for your budget. I mean, there have been times when that has been my experience too. But my challenge to you is to be sure that is true rather than just making assumptions. Research and investigate your options. Dare to go out of your way and take some time to find what you might be able to do more affordably while living within your means.

Maybe paying higher prices for organic everything is out of the question. But could you consider prioritizing more home-cooked meals and less takeout or fast food, cooking 80 percent of meals at home? Contrary to popular belief, fast food can be more expensive than eating organic home-cooked meals.

For example, I recently learned that one fast-food meal (such as a Whopper, fries, some sauce, and a drink from Burger King) would cost more than fifteen dollars as of late 2024. *For one person.* No, really, go on their website and put those items in your online cart to see for yourself. I'm sure that by the time you read this, it may cost even more than that. On the contrary, I could go to Whole Foods Market (also known as one of the most expensive grocery stores on the planet) and buy organic chicken breast, organic potatoes, and organic broccoli that would make two home-cooked meals for about twenty dollars, which breaks down to ten dollars per meal.

The good news is that, generally, it is possible to eat healthier meals affordably. Whether that's choosing a less expensive grocery store, picking up from local farms, or using a resource such as Azure Standard to source higher-quality food staples, it can be done with a little added effort. Convenience is often touted as cheaper, but it comes with a cost too—to our wallets and well-being. We pay for speed and ease, whether it's fast food or delivery, one way or another.

On the other hand, we also pay for quality, usually with our time or by sacrificing some of the convenience we have grown so accustomed to culturally. That is why we have to ask ourselves, Is it *always* more expensive to choose healthy options? Or is it just less convenient?

Of course, there are plenty of healthy things that truly are expensive: fancy treatments, gym memberships, Apple Watches, and other popular gadgets. But getting back to nature—to the way God designed us to live, even if just by 1 or 2 percent at a time—doesn't require all those fancy things. It simply requires being thoughtful about what we fuel our bodies with, how we use our time, and where we spend our money. So let's avoid the mistake of not making any inconvenient investments into our health before actually investigating what we *can* do.

And don't compare how much you can do with how much someone else who's in a different tax bracket can do. God isn't asking you to keep up with the Joneses, not even in the area of health. But He does call you to be a good and faithful steward of what has been entrusted to *you*. Just some food for thought (pun totally intended).

BE A PIPELINE, NOT A BUCKET

Years ago, I spoke at a small-church event and after my presentation, the pastor got up onstage and shared a brief lesson on stewardship that I think is worth sharing as we navigate the tension of being wise stewards of both our bodies and our money.

"Be a pipeline, not a bucket," he said.

He used this visual to explain that when it comes to the resources God gives us—our time, talents, money, bodies, energy, and so on—it's not supposed to *stop* with us. Those resources and tools are given to us to help us fulfill our callings and should flow through us freely and generously, as if flowing through a pipeline.

As a reminder, stewardship requires a heart posture with open hands that says, "Everything I have is Yours, God." So we have to shift from viewing the money we have as ours to instead viewing it as God's, which means we bring our financial decisions before Him and ultimately use our finances to bless others and bring Him glory. Donating to a charity or the needy is one way to do that. We also do bless others when we invest those resources wisely, whether that's into a physical asset (such as a piece of property), into our families, or into our physical bodies.

Am I saying that spending money on yourself—on your health—can be godly? Yes.

Doesn't that just make you a bucket? If you're using it for yourself? Not necessarily.

So many Christians have believed the lie that it's vain to spend money on their health. In reality, spending on or investing in our well-being is not inherently selfish or wrong. In fact, sometimes spending money is necessary to steward our health well. If we invest in our health *so that* we have the energy and vitality we need to fulfill our callings to the very best of our ability, that's quite different from just frivolously or selfishly spending money on something we don't need.

Think about it: If my body is not well nourished, rested, and hydrated—if I'm dealing with imbalance or symptoms that an unhealthy environment or diet may contribute to—I may do a pretty crummy job when it comes to the roles God has given me to fill and the people He has put in front of me to serve. I'm not as patient or nurturing as I would like to be for my family, I'm not as creative in my writing, and I'm not as organized and disciplined as I know I could be because I'm drained from dealing with symptoms like mood swings and low energy.

It all begins with the body. When I don't steward my body well, it is that much harder to steward anything well. When I give my body the bare minimum and ask it to run on fumes instead of proper fuel, I'm at such a disadvantage when it comes to doing with excellence the important work God has given me to do. And I'd be willing to bet the same is true for you too.

So, going back to the pipeline/bucket analogy, when done prayerfully and with wisdom (not randomly or thoughtlessly), investing our time and treasure into supporting our bodies is not automatically selfish or vain. It's an investment into our callings and, therefore, into eternity.

BEING GOOD TO YOUR BODY IS AN INVESTMENT INTO YOUR CALLING

Okay, so if we can agree that making wise investments into your health is not simply about glorifying yourself but is actually an investment into your calling, then being good to your body includes being wise about how and on what you spend your money.

It's seeking out the best quality while living within your means, even if it's not the most convenient thing. It's partnering with God, allowing the resources and tools He blesses you with—from your body to your money—to function like a pipeline, not a bucket. It's prayerfully inviting Him into the decisions you make regarding your physical and financial health and asking where He may be inviting you to make an investment, cut back spending, or reallocate funds.

And honestly? It's examining where we're neglecting doing the everyday free things—the disciplines that don't cost an arm and a leg. I think we spend so much time focusing on how expensive health tools and treatments may be out of our reach, completely forgetting that some of the healthiest things we can do are free.

So before complaining about how expensive red-light therapy or a top-shelf nontoxic product or healthy food delivery is, we need to ask ourselves these questions: *Am I even doing the free things? Am I prioritizing basic disciplines that aren't going to bankrupt me?* You know, things like gentle movement daily, getting more sunlight than blue light, eating breakfast instead of relying on caffeine for energy, stretching, breathing deeply, cooking meals at home, spending time in nature, plugging into a community, reading instead of scrolling, and hydrating.

We were never asked to do it all. The pressure to be a purist—someone who lives 100 percent toxin-free and uses all clean products, never touches unfiltered water, and eats only completely organic—is not pressure that comes from God.

All the gadgets, gizmos, and tools that can help us cultivate healthier environments are helpful and amazing, but God

> Stop comparing and start doing what you can to be good to *your* body—where you are, with what you have.

is still sovereign over everything we may like to do but that may be outside our means.

Remember, no one asked you to do all the same things as someone else. The only person putting the pressure on you to keep up with them is *you*. God asked you to steward only what *you* have been given—to be faithful with what *you* have.

So you can take the pressure off yourself.

I promise you'll be so much healthier when you spend less time comparing yourself to someone with a different financial situation than you and actually do just what God has asked *you* to do. There will always be someone with a little more than you, and there will always be someone with a little less than you, so stop comparing and start doing what you can to be good to *your* body—where you are, with what you have.

Our job is to prayerfully do the best we can, even if the investment we make is primarily of our time, to go out of our way for better quality during a season of life. That's all God asks of us. That's what stewardship looks like. If we are not faithfully stewarding the physical bodies we've been given to the best of our ability when our finances are small, we are foolish to think we will steward them well when we have more. Luke 16:10 says, "One who is faithful in a very little is also faithful in much." Just because we can't do *everything* doesn't mean we shouldn't do *anything*.

Just because we can't do *everything* doesn't mean we shouldn't do *anything*.

So we have to start where we are, with what we have. We have to do the foundational, free things first. We have to be willing to be inconvenienced now and then to prioritize quality and be thoughtful about where we invest our hard-earned money. It may not be easy, but it is part of how we can be good to our bodies.

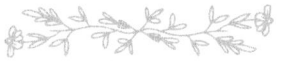

PRAYER

Thank You for the resources You have entrusted to me, God. I know that You are the provider of everything I have, from my physical body to my finances. I want to be a good manager and to steward those things well. And I know that spending financial resources on my health and well-being is more than a frivolous expense but instead is an investment. I ask for wisdom and clarity on the investments I need to make into my well-being so I can carry out my calling well. Show me which investments You are asking me to prioritize in this season and which can wait, and help me have the willingness of the Proverbs 31 woman to go out of my way to find the best quality I can within my means. Amen.

PRACTICAL APPLICATION

Consider making "wellness investments" a line item in your budget or slowly creating a wellness fund. That might look like setting aside a certain amount each month or from each paycheck into a little savings account that you earmark specifically for investments you want to make into your health, whether that's sourcing organically raised produce that costs more than conventional, investing in a water filter for your home, or something else. Setting funds aside can reduce the stress surrounding the cost of some of the things you want to prioritize and can help bring more clarity to deciding which health-related investments you should make financially.

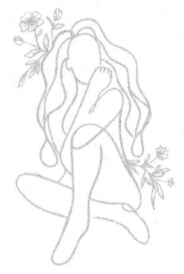

Chapter 16

DON'T WORRY, BE HEALTHY

You know what is so frustrating? When you try to do all the right things and yet things still go wrong.

Here's what I mean: In the first half of my twenties, I tried to make good decisions in my life. I worked hard to get to a stable place financially. I got married and settled down. I tried to eat healthily, although there was a lot I had to learn and unlearn about what "eating healthy" meant. But then I had pregnancy loss after pregnancy loss and I couldn't understand why that kept happening.

Then when I finally was able to carry a pregnancy, I did everything I could to prepare for the most natural birth possible, yet the delivery was quite traumatic. A baby born three weeks before his due date and an unplanned C-section later, I was over the moon and so grateful to finally have a live birth. At the same time, I kind of felt that I barely stumbled over that finish line and I couldn't help but think that my body kind of stunk at the whole pregnancy thing.

Again, I felt as though I had done everything right—nourished my body in pregnancy, rested as much as possible, read books and took classes and hired a doula for birth—yet my plans went sideways and the actions I'd taken to prepare seemed pretty pointless.

My birth plan, which had failed, and every one of those miscarriages were jarring for me because they shook me of any sense of entitlement and control I thought I had.

Entitlement? Yes. While not fun to admit, I think there was a part of me (call it my pride) that believed I *deserved* good things (like children) because I tried to do the "right" things.

Boy, did God humble me. When I was experiencing miscarriages, I was entitled and prideful in thinking, *I don't deserve this.* And then when He graciously gave us a double portion (two sons in the same year, through both adoption and birth), I thought about all the bitterness I had admittedly held toward God over the years prior—the ones riddled with grief, doubt, and hard questions. And I had that same feeling of *I don't deserve this,* but this time from a place of awe and humility.

> God doesn't give according to what I deserve. He gives according to His grace—grace upon endless grace.

Through that journey, I learned that God doesn't give according to what I deserve. He gives according to His grace—grace upon endless grace.

And the illusion of control? I struggled with that too. On the one hand, loss showed me how little control I truly have over most things—even the most important things, like my children's lives—and on the other hand, it made me want to reach for control in any way I possibly could.

Sometimes when it seems as though life is spinning out of control, when our hearts get broken or we experience trauma that we didn't sign up for, we begin to grasp at straws (at least I know I do, even if I don't intend to). What might begin as an attempt to solve problems, create better disciplines, or improve our lives in some way (such as improving our health) can spiral into extreme, self-imposed restrictions and rules to live by, which give a sense of control. It feels comfortable and peaceful to have something we can manage when the circumstances around us feel like chaos.

But the irony is that when a health journey is driven by a need for control, what may begin as a well-intended attempt to implement healthy habits can quickly spin *out* of control. Before we know it, the rules, restrictions, and protocols begin to control *us*.

That is why we have to be on guard. If we put our hope in the health stuff (the food, the workouts, the clean products, the macro tracking), we will absolutely crumble when those things don't yield the results we expect—when we make all the healthy choices and do all the right things, but things still go wrong.

All the green juice, red lights, detoxes, air filtration, organic food, supplements, and workouts in the world can't save us; only Jesus can. Those are all good things, but we must be careful not to turn good things into god things.

As good as our choices may be, we still live in a fallen world, and the best things the world has to offer are weak gods that will always let us down. All the green juice, red lights, detoxes, air filtration, organic food, supplements, and workouts in the world can't save us; only Jesus can. Those are all good things, but be careful not to turn good things into god things.

OUT OF CONTROL

It was after midnight. Should I have been sleeping? Yes. Was I? No. What was I doing? I was staring into the blue light of my phone, deep down a research rabbit hole. Maybe I was reading about the problem with food dyes and how to spot non-food ingredients in products sold as food, why it's not good to drink hot coffee out of to-go cups because microplastics affect fertility, the benefit of beef liver and organ meats, or how to heal one's microbiome.

I honestly couldn't even tell you what I was looking up because these late-night research rabbit holes happened often early on in my health journey. I was a sponge and wanted to soak up as much knowledge as I could. And knowledge is power, right? I was awakened to the dangers of so much that I'd long accepted as safe and healthy, from genetically modified food to medical system norms to toxins in products.

By learning more about those types of things, the knowledge I gained seemed to give me a bit of power back. As I became more aware of not only my body and its biological needs but also the world around me, I felt empowered to think twice before just accepting conventional methods and instead to look for more natural and healthy alternatives and make better decisions.

And I'm thankful for that. That is a gift. But I'd be remiss if I didn't admit that some of the ways I learned or responded to those realities were far from healthy. For one thing, I was sacrificing one of my most basic needs—sleep—as I found a thousand things to worry about. I'm sure that was just great for my cortisol. No wonder that DUTCH test revealed that my adrenals were shot.

The more I learned, the longer my list of "rules to be healthy" grew. They really should have been guidelines—things to be aware of and minimize or prioritize where and when possible. But no, for a little while at the beginning of my journey, they were hard-and-fast restrictions.

No dairy.

No gluten.

No soy.

No toxins.

No caffeine.

No plastic.

No EMFs.

No seed oils.

No . . . *fun*.

Listen, I was the oldest child in my family, a type A personality, and a strict rule follower. So when a rule is set, you won't catch me breaking it. Maybe you can relate. Anyway, I thought I was being healthy. I was healing my body and fertility, right?

Kind of. Yes, making some of those changes was absolutely beneficial for my well-being, and some have become a normal part of my lifestyle now. But there were times along the way when I was kind of miserable and felt burdened by it all. I had so many supplements to take, protocols to follow, bad things to avoid, and rules to keep that I really wasn't living. Having knowledge and awareness is one thing, but trying to avoid every unhealthy thing—the brokenness of the world, really—is a heavy burden to shoulder on your own.

> While diet culture is toxic, anti-diet culture can be just as toxic.

WHAT DOES REAL FREEDOM LOOK LIKE?

Please don't mishear me. I'm not saying life should just be a free-for-all with no limitations on the desires of our flesh, like drinking to oblivion or eating a whole cake. Self-control is biblical.

And while diet culture is toxic, anti-diet culture can be just as toxic when it swings too far into the opposite extreme, where the mindset for things like carbs and calories turns into "anything goes" in the name of food freedom.

Let me be clear: True freedom does not mean a free-for-all.

I love this analogy by Tim Keller: "Because a fish absorbs oxygen from water, not air, it's free only if it's restricted to water. If a fish is 'freed' from the river and put out on the grass to explore, its freedom to move and soon live is destroyed. Real freedom isn't restrictionless, it's finding the right ones."[1]

Some rules, or guidelines and limitations, are actually necessary for freedom; there are bounds in which we are created to thrive. When we cast away any and all limitations, we can drive ourselves into destruction.

So I'm not suggesting that all rules are burdens. Some guidelines and restrictions—like drinking enough water, spending adequate time outside, and minimizing eating food-like products devoid of nutrients—actually help us thrive.

Rules become burdensome and sometimes even harmful when they are rooted in fear and restrict us from the very things that contribute to our thriving. For example, when we say no to enjoyment and community (something that is critical to our human design and well-being) every time we are invited simply because we're afraid the food at a restaurant may not be cooked in the healthiest oils, is that actually *healthy*? I think not.

MAYBE YOU JUST NEED A NAP AND A SNACK

Remember, Proverbs 17:22 says that "a cheerful heart is *good medicine*" (NIV, emphasis added). Yes, nutritious food and fresh air and movement are good medicine, of course. But what about wearing your favorite dress and dancing the night away? A laugh with loved ones? A perfectly brewed cup of coffee or extra-frothy cappuccino? Sleeping in and making pancakes on Saturday? The little joys that can make life feel a little lighter in an otherwise hard and heavy world? Those things are good medicine too—according to the Bible, anyway.

Science confirms that. Researchers of a Johns Hopkins University study found that "a general sense of well-being—feeling cheerful, relaxed, energetic, and satisfied with life—actually reduces the chances of a heart attack."[2]

Why are we not talking about that more?

Instead of obsessing over the next fad diet or magic potion or gut protocol, maybe we should be asking, *Did I laugh today?* Think about it. When was the last time you took a deep breath and felt content? Took a nap? Read a good book? Had a snack?

Really, we're all just basically older versions of kids. And maybe your hormones aren't totally out of whack. Maybe you just need a nap and a (nourishing) snack.

Kidding. Kind of.

I'm not saying that's all there is to health, but I am saying that sometimes it really is that simple and basic. Rest, sleep, nourish your body—and then go do the things God made you to do.

Think of Elijah in the Bible in 1 Kings 19. He talked to God and essentially said, "I quit and would rather be dead" (see verse 4). He was burned-out, so God took him to a resting place beneath a fig tree. (I love that, because figs are actually so nutrient dense and are packed with good things like fiber, copper, potassium, magnesium, manganese, calcium, and vitamin K.[3] But I digress.)

Anyway, God told Elijah to sleep and provided food for him to eat. After that, Elijah was ready for ministry—to fulfill the call on his life—again. Nap and a snack—it's simple *and* it's biblical.

I think the question we have to ask ourselves, then, is, How do we know if our pursuit of health has become unhealthy? I've found that if I answer no to either of the following questions, I have crossed the line to unhealthy: *Is this new habit, discipline, or lifestyle change* supporting *my calling or* suffocating *it? Is it helping me feel better, show up with my energy, and fulfill the roles God has given me, or is it causing me stress and becoming a distraction from what actually matters?*

That's the line. And the details of that will look different for every one of us because we each have different circumstances, support systems, seasons of life, and capacities. But we have to run every new discipline or change we make through this lens: *Is it making me a better disciple of Jesus in whatever role I hold [wife, mom, teacher], or is it making me miserable to be around?*

There have been times when prioritizing my health has absolutely made me a better version of myself, which is what getting healthy should do. However, there have also been times when I've gotten carried away.

I remember one time my husband came home from the store and said, "I got some low-fat Greek yogur—," and before he could finish, I cut him off and proceeded to ramble on about all that I had recently learned about low-fat dairy versus whole-fat dairy.

After giving him an entire science lesson to my satisfaction, he looked at me with the most deadpan face and said, "Babe, I barely got six words out before you gave me an entire expository essay I didn't ask for."

And that, my friend, is an example of a time when I realized I was way too far over the line. I was becoming miserable to be around. My research and interest in making the healthiest choices possible were no longer making me a better wife and helpmate. Frankly, I was becoming quite annoying.

YOU CAN'T HEAL YOURSELF

Wait just a minute. What do I mean, "You can't heal yourself"? Isn't that the entire thesis, the whole selling point, of the wellness industry? And don't we believe our bodies are designed to be able to heal? If our hormones have gone haywire or we're dealing with chronic illness or disease or something else, isn't it possible to heal if we find and address root causes?

Yup—to a point.

God *did* design our bodies intelligently, and they have an innate ability to heal and repair. The body often *can* heal when it's given what it needs: good, God-made things. Pretty cool, huh?

While the body's ability to heal is true and amazing, we might take that to mean that all healing is on us. It's completely up to us what *we* partake in: the food we eat, the supplements we take, the habits and disciplines we implement, and the products we use. If we can heal ourselves, what do we need God for?

We've already established that those things *do* matter, but God also called Himself the Great Physician. Although He seemed to be using that as a metaphor in reference to spiritual sickness, I'd argue that it applies to physical ailments too.

I mean, look at all the miracles Jesus performed in the Gospels. From healing a leper to a woman who had been bleeding for years. They were healed because of their faith and because it was God's will, not because they biohacked their way to restoration. Healing began in their hearts before it touched their physical bodies: They believed Jesus was sovereign and that He could do what all the best things on earth could not. Now that's not to say God always heals because of faith. There are plenty of faithful people who do not experience complete physical healing on this side of heaven, but the point is that it's ultimately up to His sovereignty, not our striving.

Plus, if we put the full burden of healing on our decisions, choices, and lifestyles, it can create what feels like an existential crisis when healing does not happen how we expect or breakdown still occurs. Because, yes, in an ideal world—or in an Edenic world, the world we were originally made for—our bodies should be able to heal and repair themselves 100 percent of the time.

But we don't live in an Edenic world anymore; we live in a world marred by sin, which means disease, decay, and death touch us on this side of heaven. We may not always experience full physical healing, even with the purest, healthiest lifestyle we could imagine.

God does invite us to participate in our well-being, though. He gave us choices, and it doesn't take a rocket scientist to know that some of those choices will benefit our well-being and others will harm it. So, again, what we do or don't do *does* matter.

However, if we put the burden of healing on ourselves, we cut God—the creator of our bodies—out of the equation entirely. We are invited to partner with God in caring for the bodies He gave us, doing the best we can and trusting Him to be sovereign over it all instead of shouldering a burden that was never ours to carry.

Although I focus on the things I can control, such as the skin care I choose to use or what food I eat as fuel, there are so many things outside my control—things I don't even know about that I really do have to entrust to the Lord.

I can't help but think of my toddlers when I say that. They are so excited about life, exploring the world around them. If they're paying attention, they manage to avoid running into the corner of my dining room table. But most of the time, they are fixated on the toys they are playing with or whatever else has their attention, and I often put my hand on the corner of the table just before one of them bonks his head on it.

My little mom reflexes protect them. They don't get hurt, so they don't stop running about. They just keep going, blissfully unaware that the corner of the table—a hazard that could have harmed them—was even there at all.

It's humbling to think how many times God has probably protected me from something hazardous that I didn't even know was there as I went about my life. How arrogant would it be to think I alone am in control of my healing and all that could affect my body?

The bottom line is this: You can't heal yourself. You are not God. But you *can* decide how you'll steward your health. You can diligently support the body He so intelligently crafted to repair, heal, and thrive when it lives aligned with His design.

And although your best efforts and even all the best things of this world may not be able to heal every possible thing that could go wrong, you *can* be an example to all believers of what it means to treat your body like a temple of the Holy Spirit and daughter of the King: in how you live, move, eat, and be.

BEING GOOD TO YOUR BODY IS . . .

With all that in mind, what does being good to your body look like?

Practically speaking, it might look like living what some call an 80/20 lifestyle. That might involve having a diet made of 80 percent healthy, whole foods and 20 percent foods that may not have the best ingredients or cleanest labels. The 20 percent buffer is meant to add a sense of realistic wiggle room, since being able to live 100 percent perfectly healthy is far from likely. The 80/20 lifestyle maintains a sense of discipline while allowing for grace and flexibility—like eating dinner at a popular restaurant with friends or ordering a yummy dessert—without guilt or fear.

Are you doing those not-so-healthy things every day, all the time? No. But occasionally? In moderation? Totally. Go for it. That 80/20 concept is basically meant to represent discipline with moderation.

But not everyone will start off with an 80/20 split right off the bat. For example, when you first begin a health journey, your ratio might look more like 20/80.

You may have plenty of lifestyle shifts to make and habits to create, and you may be starting off closer to 100 percent not-so-healthy ones. Do you need to change 80 percent overnight? No. You could, however, change maybe 10 percent, such as by making a handful of swaps to reduce your toxin exposure. Then, with time, you might make a few more changes that bring you to 20 percent better than you were.

So, is 80/20 what some might consider the goal? Representative of discipline with moderation, or what some might call a balanced approach? Probably. Somewhere around there anyway. Maybe 80/20, 90/10, or 70/30. I'm not trying to math my entire life and would rather not revisit learning fractions. But the point is that the goal, on

> Being good to your body requires the right heart posture. It is trusting that God is God and you are not. It is partnering with Him on a health or healing journey. It is releasing the burden to heal yourself to the One who holds it all.

a practical level, looks like working toward making choices that align with the good things God designed for us to thrive the *ma-*

jority of the time (but no perfection required, because that's not possible). And, of course, there may be a season you need to be more strict and others when you have to be more flexible.

Biblically speaking, you must trust God rather than all the things that create worry. And it ultimately still comes back to the posture of stewardship: "Everything I have is Yours, God." It's saying, "My body, my time, my resources? All of these things are Yours. I will take utmost care of my body because of the gift that it is. I will spend my time wisely; I won't take for granted a single minute or breath I'm given. And I will use the resources You entrust to me—including my body—to live a life worthy of the calling" (see Ephesians 4:1–6).

Being good to your body requires the right heart posture. It is trusting that God is God and you are not. It is partnering with Him on a health or healing journey. It is releasing the burden to heal yourself to the One who holds it all. And it's a cheerful heart—finding joy and whimsy and fun in the everyday, not just putting yourself in a health prison, afraid of the world around you. Because a cheerful heart is good medicine.

A cheerful heart is a heart that is light because it is not burdened by the weight of trying to control everything around you, because you trust the One who holds the world in His hands.

LIVE A LITTLE

After a period of time living quite strictly in an effort to reduce inflammation and heal root causes, I heard a sermon on idolatry and it convicted me. I realized that somewhere along the way, that's what health, natural living, my healing journey—whatever you want to call it—was becoming to me. And I knew it was time to change some things. I didn't go crazy and throw in the towel altogether (because that isn't healthy either), but I did go out to eat with some girlfriends, share a pizza, stay past closing, and could not. stop. laughing. And that felt more therapeutic and life-giving for me than fancy supplements and treatments or avoiding every possible red-flag ingredient.

It makes sense, really. If we look at the body holistically, we know that it is affected not just by what we do physically but also by our mental, spiritual, and relational well-being. And if the pursuit of physical health regularly bulldozes or harms any of those three aspects, that will eventually create elevated levels of stress and inevitably have negative repercussions for the body.

Let's definitely try *not* to willingly lather our bodies in harmful chemicals, eat tons of food-like products that are actually made of non-food, or live super-stagnant lifestyles, because those things aren't good for our bodies. But let's also not bend over backward to avoid every last toxin, miss moments with our family because we just can't skip a workout, or stay away from social gatherings because eating out isn't the healthiest. Perhaps that may be necessary for a short period of time for healing, but it's not healthy as a lifestyle. Avoiding those things altogether out of fear also isn't good for us, because it's not good for our minds (and our brains are literally part of our bodies).

There's a middle ground here, and it *always* comes back to stewardship.

That should be the truth that anchors us and guides every decision. Our decisions do hold weight, but stewardship means giving our bodies the best we can and trusting that the creator of our bodies is bigger than the brokenness of the world we live in and sovereign over all.

So, to recap, are all restrictions bad? Of course not. Self-control and caring for our bodies well is biblical. It matters.

But as with anything, when rules shift from guidelines for being good to the bodies God gave us to trying to control, fix, manipulate, or even heal our bodies on our own accord, that's when we can slip into idolatry and when things can get pretty unhealthy.

So yes, take good care of your body, because it's a good gift, not a project to fix. Trust that the God who stitched you together is sovereign over every little thing—every breath you take and every fiber of your being.

Don't worry, be healthy, and give the glory to the giver of every good and perfect gift by being good to your fearfully and wonderfully made body.

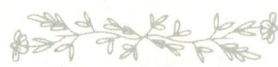

PRAYER

God, I want to be good to my body. I want to be the best steward of the vessel You gave me that I can possibly be, without stumbling into the burden of relying on myself for everything and without getting tangled up in fear and worry. I know I fail to find the balance daily. I know there are times I don't care for my body the way I should, either neglecting to do the basic things or going overboard and obsessing over everything. Help me remember that living healthfully and supporting my body is a means to an end—to fulfill my calling and bring You glory—not the end itself. I know that I can live life fully only when I trust You fully. So here I am, placing my health, body, and whole life in Your hands. And I will continue to do so over and over again. Everything I have is Yours, Lord. Amen.

PRACTICAL APPLICATION

If you are in a season of taking your health very seriously, perhaps even being too controlling, pick one thing you will do this week to have fun and live a little more fully, without stress or worry, to bring some balance to your life. Can you plan a girls' brunch at a local café you love? Or maybe have a family pizza night?

On the other hand, if you're in a season where you have not been focusing on or prioritizing your health, pick one proactive step you will take to practice more self-control. Can you back off from that whole bag of chocolate chips you've been eating before bed, maybe eating only a handful or switching to a more nourishing snack? Or cut back on caffeine, screen time, or something else that is inhibiting your thriving?

Decide one thing you will shift, and commit to implementing it *this week*. Ask someone you love, such as your spouse or a friend, to hold you accountable and help you see it through.

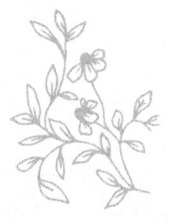

LABEL-READING CHEAT SHEET

ITEM	HOW TO SPOT IT ON A LABEL
Fragrance or Perfume	fragrance, perfume, parfum, aroma
Ethoxylated Ingredients	PPG, PEG, polysorbate, and words ending in -*eth* like laureth, steareth, and ceteareth
Ethanolamine Compounds	triethanolamine (TEA), diethanolamine (DEA), cocamide DEA, cocamide MEA, DEA-cetyl phosphate, DEA-oleth-3 phosphate, lauramide DEA, linoleamide MEA, myristamide DEA, oleamide DEA, stearamide MEA, TEA-lauryl sulfate
Butylated Compounds (BHA and BHT)	butylated hydroxyanisole (BHA), butylated hydroxytoluene (BHT)
Parabens	ethylparaben, butylparaben, benzylparaben, isobutylparaben, methylparaben, isopropylparaben, propylparaben
Formaldehyde-Releasing Preservatives	DMDM hydantoin, diazolidinyl urea, imidazolidinyl urea, glyoxal, sodium hydroxymethylglycinate, quaternium-15, 2-bromo-2-nitropropane-1,3-diol

CONCERN

According to the Campaign for Safe Cosmetics, dozens, sometimes even hundreds, of chemicals can hide under one little word—*fragrance*—on the product labels of the beauty and personal-care products you use every day. Some are known endocrine disruptors, allergens, and carcinogens.[1]

They are a group of ingredients made by the process of ethoxylation. This manufacturing process can result in two toxic contaminants, ethylene oxide and 1,4-dioxane, which have been linked to health concerns such as cancer.[2]

They may break down in the product and form carcinogenic N-nitroso compounds (NOCs). Possible concerns are skin irritation, asthma or difficulty breathing if inhaled in large quantities, and damage to fertility and/or unborn child.[3]

BHA is a preservative that is often used in cosmetics, especially in lipstick and eye shadow. It has been added as a carcinogen to the "State of California's Proposition 65 List of Chemicals Known to the State to Cause Cancer or Reproductive Toxicity," and studies show some endocrine-disrupting effects. BHT is a preservative that is often used in food and personal-care products. Concerns include hormone disruption, allergies, and carcinogenic impact.[4]

Paraben preservatives are associated with disruption of the endocrine (hormone) system.[5]

These preservatives release a small amount of formaldehyde into a product over time. The International Agency for Research on Cancer (IARC) has classified formaldehyde as "carcinogenic to humans."[6]

ITEM	HOW TO SPOT IT ON A LABEL
IPBC	iodopropynyl butylcarbamate
Phenoxyethanol	phenoxyethanol (PhE), 2- phenoxyethanol
Phthalates	DEP, DBP, DEHP, fragrance
Synthetic Dyes/Pigments	Blue 1 Lake, Red 40 Lake, Red 6 Lake, Red 6, FD&C Red 40 (CI 16035), FD&C Yellow 5 (CI 19140)
Petroleum-Based Ingredients	petrolatum, petroleum jelly, paraffin oil, mineral oil
PTFE	polytetrafluoroethylene (PTFE), Teflon, polyperfluoromethylisopropyl ether, DEA-C8-18, perfluoroalkylethyl phosphate
Talc	talcum powder, cosmetic talc
Retinol	retinol, vitamin A, retinyl acetate, retinyl palmitate, all-trans retinoic acid, tretinoin
Aluminum Hydroxide	aluminum hydroxide

CONCERN

It may cause dermal irritation or contact allergy. It is also toxic to the lungs when inhaled so should be avoided in products that can be inhaled.[7]

The American Contact Dermatitis Society (ACDS) lists it as one of its core allergens, even in concentrations as low as 1 percent.[8]

This includes a large group of chemicals, including dibutyl phthalate (DBP), diethylhexyl phthalate (DEHP), diethyl phthalate (DEP), dimethyl phthalate (DMP), and butyl benzyl phthalate (BBP). Endocrine disruption, developmental and reproductive toxicity, and cancer are health concerns linked to phthalates.[9]

May have the residues of carcinogenic (cancer-causing) and endocrine-disrupting by-products of petroleum. These are commonly used in colored beauty products such as lipstick.

Often found in such beauty products as lotion and makeup, the primary concern is that they can be contaminated with polycyclic aromatic hydrocarbons (PAHs), many of which have been considered possible carcinogens.[10]

Polytetrafluoroethylene (PTFE) is more commonly known as Teflon. It has been associated with endocrine disruption and cancer.[11]

Talc may contain the known carcinogen asbestos. Health concerns include irritation, cancer, and respiratory toxicity.[12]

Retinol derivatives, in combination with sunlight, may increase the risk of skin cancer.[13]

Elemental aluminum is controversial, as it is linked to Alzheimer's disease. Additionally, it is a pro-oxidant and can increase the potential for oxidative skin damage.[14]

ITEM	HOW TO SPOT IT ON A LABEL
Chemical UV Filters	octinoxate, homosalate, octisalate, octocrylene, avobenzone
Lead and Heavy Metals	(not listed on labels)

CONCERN

Concerns include endocrine disruption, allergic reaction, and possible damage to an unborn child.[15]

Heavy metals such as lead, arsenic, and cadmium (often found in the makeup pigments and dyes used in cosmetics) are not listed on the labels because they are contaminants, not ingredients. The best way to avoid levels of heavy metals that exceed European or Canadian limits is to research and purchase from trustworthy makeup companies that source high-purity/quality makeup pigments and have protocols in place to minimize heavy metal levels (such as third-party testing).[16]

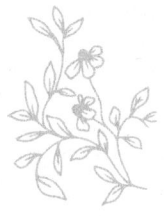

ACKNOWLEDGMENTS

My husband and best friend, Matt: Thank you for all the ways you have supported me through this project, from taking the kids to give me time to work when inspiration struck to helping me think through ideas and listening to my late-night brainstorm sessions. This would not have been possible without your belief in me and unending support. Also, thank you for coming up with the perfect title for this book. All title credit goes to you!

Mom and Dad: Thank you for all the support and love you've shown me over the past several years, not only as I worked on this book but also through my health journey during all the years prior to writing a single word. You have been some of my biggest cheerleaders in every season and through every endeavor, and there will never be enough thank-yous for that.

My editor, Susan, and the entire Penguin Random House team: Thank you for believing in me all these years, guiding me through every project, and helping shape me into a better and more confident writer with each project we work on together. I truly believe this is our best one yet, and I have your consistent feedback and mentorship to thank for that!

My literary agent, Bryan: Thank you for being more than just an agent but also a true friend to me and our family. Your support through every step of the publishing process is a gift, and your friendship is a treasure. Grateful is an understatement.

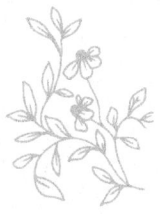

NOTES

Chapter 1: How Did We Get Here?

1. Nancy R. Pearcey, *Love Thy Body: Answering Hard Questions About Life and Sexuality* (Baker Books, 2018), 21.

2. Pearcey, *Love Thy Body,* 24.

3. Elisabeth Elliot, "The Discipline of the Body, Part Two," ElisabethElliot.org, June 30, 2022, https://elisabethelliot.org/resource-library/devotionals/the-discipline-of-the-body-part-two.

4. Dan Witters, "U.S. Depression Rates Reach New Highs," Gallup, May 17, 2023, https://news.gallup.com/poll/505745/depression-rates-reach-new-highs.aspx.

5. Gabriel A. Benavidez et al., "Chronic Disease Prevalence in the US: Sociodemographic and Geographic Variations by Zip Code Tabulation Area," *Preventing Chronic Disease* 21, February 29, 2024, http://dx.doi.org/10.5888/pcd21.230267.

6. Joel Achenbach et al., "An Epidemic of Chronic Illness Is Killing Us Too Soon," *The Washington Post,* October 3, 2023,

www.washingtonpost.com/health/interactive/2023/american
-life-expectancy-dropping.

Chapter 2: Where Are We Going Wrong?

1. "Autoimmune Diseases," National Institute of Environmental Health Sciences, last reviewed April 23, 2025, www.niehs.nih.gov/health/topics/conditions/autoimmune.

2. Julia Evangelou Strait, "Breast Cancer Rates Increasing Among Younger Women," WashU Medicine, January 26, 2024, https://medicine.wustl.edu/news/breast-cancer-rates-increasing-among-younger-women.

3. M. Ashraf Ganie and Sanjay Kalra, "Polycystic Ovary Syndrome—A Metabolic Malady, the Mother of All Lifestyle Disorders in Women—Can Indian Health Budget Tackle It in Future?," *Indian Journal of Endocrinology and Metabolism* 15, no. 4 (October–December 2011): 239–41, https://pmc.ncbi.nlm.nih.gov/articles/PMC3193771.

4. "General Information/Press Room," American Thyroid Association, www.thyroid.org/media-main/press-room.

5. "Health and Well-Being," Status of Women in the States, https://statusofwomendata.org/explore-the-data/health-well-being.

6. Mary N. Woessner et al., "The Evolution of Technology and Physical Inactivity: The Good, the Bad, and the Way Forward," *Frontiers in Public Health* 9 (May 2021), https://doi.org/10.3389/fpubh.2021.655491.

7. Bernard Srour et. al, "Ultra-Processed Food Intake and Risk of Cardiovascular Disease: Prospective Cohort Study (NutriNet-Santé)," *BMJ* (2019), https://doi.org/10.1136/bmj.l1451.

8. Jacinta Lowes and Marika Tiggemann, "Body Dissatisfaction, Dieting Awareness and the Impact of Parental Influence in

Young Children," *British Journal of Health Psychology* 8, no. 2 (May 2003): 135–47, https://doi.org/10.1348/13591070 3321649123.

9. Natalie Schreyer, "Most Medical Research Is Done on Men. That's a Deadly Problem," *Mother Jones*, July 21, 2016, www .motherjones.com/environment/2016/07/men-women-health -inquiring-minds; Jana Plevkova et al., "Various Aspects of Sex and Gender Bias in Biomedical Research," *Physiological Research* 69, no. 3 (December 2020): 367–78, www.ncbi.nlm .nih.gov/pmc/articles/PMC8603716; Priyanka Jain and Laine Bruzek, "In a World Built for Men, We Don't Know Much About Women's Bodies," *Fortune*, June 10, 2022, https:// fortune.com/2022/06/10/world-built-for-men-women -bodies-gender-gap-health-research-medicine-care-jain -bruzek.

10. "How Intermittent Fasting Affects Women," Cleveland Clinic, July 17, 2023, health.clevelandclinic.org/intermittent -fasting-for-women.

11. "Gonadotropin-Releasing Hormone (GnRH)," Cleveland Clinic, March 18, 2022, https://my.clevelandclinic.org/health /body/22525-gonadotropin-releasing-hormone.

12. Julia Zumpano, quoted in "How Intermittent Fasting Affects Women."

13. "Early Puberty," *PBS News Hour*, video, May 31, 2024, www .pbs.org/video/early-puberty-1717186232.

14. Alexandra M. Binder et al., "Childhood and Adolescent Phenol and Phthalate Exposure and the Age of Menarche in Latina Girls," *Environmental Health* 17, no. 32 (April 2018), https://ehjournal.biomedcentral.com/articles/10.1186/s12940 -018-0376-z.

15. Shanaz Dairkee et al., "Reduction of Daily-Use Parabens and Phthalates Reverses Accumulation of Cancer-Associated

Phenotypes Within Disease-Free Breast Tissue of Study Subjects," *Chemosphere* (May 2023), https://pubmed.ncbi.nlm.nih.gov/36746253.

16. Sujana Reddy et al., "Physiology, Circadian Rhythm," *StatPearls* (May 2023), www.ncbi.nlm.nih.gov/books/NBK 519507.

17. Alisa Vitti, "Infradian Rhythm: Your Guide to a Perfect Cycle," FLO Living, November 7, 2023, https://floliving.com /blog/infradian-rhythm.

18. Alisa Vitti, "Cycle Sync to Improve Productivity, Health, and Relationships," *SHE,* podcast, https://jordanleedooley.com /shownotes/cycle-syncing-to-improve-productivity -relationships-and-health.

Chapter 3: What Does the Bible Say?

1. Bible Study Tools, "Yare'," www.biblestudytools.com/lexicons /hebrew/nas/yare.html.

2. Lori Stanley Roeleveld, "What Does It Mean to Be 'Fearfully and Wonderfully Made'? (Psalm 139:14)," Christianity.com, October 22, 2024, www.christianity.com/wiki/bible/what -does-psalm-139-mean-fearfully-and-wonderfully-made .html.

3. Caoimhe Twohig-Bennett and Andy Jones, "The Health Benefits of the Great Outdoors: A Systematic Review and Meta-Analysis of Greenspace Exposure and Health Outcomes," *Environmental Resources* 166 (October 2018): 628–37, https://pmc.ncbi.nlm.nih.gov/articles/PMC6562165.

Chapter 5: Reframe Your Body Beliefs

1. Isabella Backman, "Endometriosis," *Yale Medicine Magazine,* spring 2024, issue 172 Women's Health Special Report, https://medicine.yale.edu/news/yale-medicine-magazine /article/endometriosis.

2. Timothy Keller, *Counterfeit Gods: The Empty Promises of Money, Sex, and Power, and the Only Hope That Matters* (Viking, 2009).

Chapter 6: Shed the Shame

1. Brené Brown, "Brené Brown on Shame and Accountability," *Unlocking Us*, podcast, July 1, 2020, https://brenebrown.com /podcast/brene-on-shame-and-accountability.

2. Robert Karen, "Shame," *The Atlantic*, February 1992, www .theatlantic.com/magazine/archive/1992/02/shame/670008.

3. Jaquelle Crowe, "Ashamed of My Body: Six Truths for Struggling Teens," *Desiring God* (blog), June 6, 2017, www .desiringgod.org/articles/ashamed-of-my-body.

4. Jess Connolly, "Breaking Free from Body Shame," *Hope Heals* (blog), accessed March 11, 2025, https://hopeheals.com /articles-archive/breaking-free-from-body-shame.

Chapter 8: Reduce Your Burden

1. "1,4-Dioxane," Campaign for Safe Cosmetics, www.safe cosmetics.org/chemicals/14-dioxane.

2. "Parabens," Campaign for Safe Cosmetics, www.safecosmetics .org/chemicals/parabens.

3. "Low-Dose Exposures," Campaign for Safe Cosmetics, www.safecosmetics.org/resources/health-science/low-dose -exposures.

4. Mayo Clinic Staff, "Stress Symptoms: Effects on Your Body and Behavior," Mayo Clinic, August 10, 2023, www.mayo clinic.org/healthy-lifestyle/stress-management/in-depth /stress-symptoms/art-20050987.

5. William Shaw et al., "Stress Effects on the Body," American Psychological Association, October 21, 2024, www.apa.org /topics/stress/body.

Chapter 9: Reclaim Your Femininity

1. Clinical Consulting Team, "What Does DUTCH Complete? Four Groups of Hormones, Metabolites, and Other Biomarkers," DUTCH, March 2, 2021, https://dutchtest .com/articles/what-does-dutch-test-4-groups-of-hormones -metabolites-other-biomarkers.

2. Abdurrahman Coskun et al., "Physiological Rhythms and Biological Variation of Biomolecules: The Road to Personalized Laboratory Medicine," *International Journal of Molecular Sciences 24*, no. 7 (March 2023), https://pmc.ncbi .nlm.nih.gov/articles/PMC10094461.

3. Ryan Pendell, "Millennials Are Burning Out," Gallup, www .gallup.com/workplace/237377/millennials-burning.aspx.

4. George Anders, "So Stressed! Women Report Bigger Burdens but See a Lot More Escapes," *LinkedIn News*, August 25, 2021, www.linkedin.com/pulse/so-stressed-women-report -bigger-burdens-see-lot-more-escapes-anders.

5. Perfeqt Team, "Male vs. Female Rhythms: Exploring the Sun and Moon Metaphor," Perfeqt, February 10, 2023, www .perfeqt.co/blog?p=male-vs-female-rhythm-exploring-the -sun-and-moon-metaphor. See also Annika Nicole (@iamannikanciole), "Female Physiology Was Not Designed for the 8-5 Grind," January 11, 2022, www.instagram.com/p /CYmwDp5psIS/?img_index=1.

6. "Male Hormone Cycle," Hormonology, www.myhormonology .com/learn/male-hormone-cycle.

7. "Luteal Phase," Cleveland Clinic, November 24, 2022, https:// my.clevelandclinic.org/health/articles/24417-luteal-phase; Jessica E. McLaughlin, "Menstrual Cycle," Merck Manual, September 2022, www.merckmanuals.com/home/women-s -health-issues/biology-of-the-female-reproductive-system /menstrual-cycle; Abby McCoy, "How Your Menstrual Cycle

Affects Your Behavior," Everyday Health, March 21, 2024, www.everydayhealth.com/womens-health/how-your -menstrual-cycle-affects-your-behavior.aspx; Dhanalakshmi K. Thiyagarajan et al., "Physiology, Menstrual Cycle," *StatPearls,* September 27, 2024, www.ncbi.nlm.nih .gov/books/NBK500020/; Andrei Marhol, "What Happens to Hormone Levels During the Menstrual Cycle?" *Flo,* November 15, 2023, https://flo.health/menstrual-cycle/health /period/hormone-levels-during-cycle.

8. Alexandra Mysoor, "How Women Can Use Monthly Periods as a Productivity Tool," *Forbes,* May 10, 2018, www.forbes .com/sites/alexandramysoor/2018/05/10/how-women-can -use-monthly-periods-as-a-productivity-tool.

Chapter 10: Embrace Your Beauty Naturally

1. "Exposures Add Up—Survey Results," Environmental Working Group, 2004, www.ewg.org/news-insights/news /2004/12/exposures-add-survey-results.

2. Marsha McCulloch, "Eleven Surprising Benefits and Uses of Myrrh Oil," Healthline, January 4, 2019, www.healthline.com /nutrition/myrrh-oil.

3. Carrie Madormo, "Benefits of Olive Oil for Your Skin," Verywell Health, September 22, 2024, www.verywellhealth .com/olive-oil-skin-benefits-5095861.

4. Jenna Fletcher, "Honey for Skin: How to Use and Side Effects," MedicalNewsToday, April 3, 2020, www.medical newstoday.com/articles/honey-for-skin.

Chapter 11: Support Your Fertility

1. Xin Grevers et al., "Cancer Incidence Attributable to the Use of Oral Contraceptives and Hormone Therapy in Alberta in 2012," *CMAJ Open* 4, no. 4 (December 2016): 754–59, https://pmc.ncbi.nlm.nih.gov/articles/PMC5173458.

2. Jennifer Roback Morse, quoted in Nancy Pearcey, *Love Thy Body: Answering Hard Questions about Life and Sexuality* (Baker Books, 2018), 74.

3. Morse, in Pearcey, *Love Thy Body*, 75.

4. Pearcey, *Love Thy Body*, 75.

5. "One in Six People Globally Affected by Infertility: WHO," World Health Organization, April 4, 2023, www.who.int /news/item/04-04-2023-1-in-6-people-globally-affected-by -infertility.

6. Bible Hub, "2032. heron or herayon," https://biblehub.com /hebrew/2032.htm.

7. "Deeper Hebrew Meanings from the Garden of Eden," Hebrewversity, www.hebrewversity.com/deeper-hebrew -meanings-garden-eden.

8. John H. Walton, "Pain in Childbearing (Hebrew Corner 8)," Zondervan Academic, October 17, 2008, https://zondervan academic.com/blog/pain-in-childbe.

Chapter 12: Nourish Your Body

1. Scott Edwards, "Sugar and the Brain," Harvard Medical School, Spring 2016, https://hms.harvard.edu/news-events /publications-archive/brain/sugar-brain.

2. Mihir N. Nakrani et al., "Physiology, Glucose Metabolism," *StatPearls*, July 17, 2023, www.ncbi.nlm.nih.gov/books/NBK 560599.

Chapter 14: Know Your Neighbors

1. Amy Novotney, "The Risks of Social Isolation," American Psychological Association, *Monitor on Psychology* 50, no. 5 (May 2019): 32, www.apa.org/monitor/2019/05/ce-corner -isolation.

2. Brenda Egolf et al., "The Roseto Effect: A Fifty-Year Comparison of Mortality Rates," *American Journal of Public Health* 82, no. 8 (August 1992): 1089–92, www.ncbi.nlm.nih .gov/pmc/articles/PMC1695733.

3. Mayo Clinic Staff, "Friendships: Enrich Your Life and Improve Your Health," Mayo Clinic, October 15, 2024, www .mayoclinic.org/healthy-lifestyle/adult-health/in-depth /friendships/art-20044860.

Chapter 15: Invest in Your Health

1. Victoria Fu and Siddharth Somaiya, quoted in Hasina Jeelani, "Why Are Clean Beauty Products More Expensive Than Their Traditional Counterparts?," *Vogue India*, February 15, 2021, www.vogue.in/beauty/content/why-are-clean-beauty-products -more-expensive-than-their-traditional-counterparts.

Chapter 16: Don't Worry, Be Healthy

1. Timothy Keller (1950–2023) (@timkellernyc), "Because a fish absorbs oxygen from water, not air, it's free only if it's restricted to water," X, November 27, 2018, https://x.com /timkellernyc/status/1067499050092687362?lang=en.

2. Hub Staff Report, "Johns Hopkins Researchers Link Positive Outlook to Reduced Heart Attack Risk," Johns Hopkins University, July 10, 2013, https://hub.jhu.edu/2013/07/10 /happy-heart-health.

3. "Four Health Benefits of Figs," Cleveland Clinic, July 3, 2024, https://health.clevelandclinic.org/benefits-of-figs.

Label-Reading Cheat Sheet

1. "Fragrance Disclosure," Campaign for Safe Cosmetics, www .safecosmetics.org/resources/health-science/fragrance -disclosure.

2. "Ethoxylated Ingredients," Campaign for Safe Cosmetics, www.safecosmetics.org/chemicals/ethoxylated-ingredients.

3. R. F. Mankes, "Studies on the Embryopathic Effects of Ethanolamine in Long-Evans Rats: Preferential Embryopathy in Pups Contiguous with Male Siblings in Utero," *Teratogenesis, Carcinogenesis, and Mutagenesis* 6, no. 5 (1986): 403–17, https://onlinelibrary.wiley.com/doi/10.1002/tcm.1770060507; "Substance Infocard: 2-Aminoethanol," European Chemicals Agency, https://echa.europa.eu/substance-information/-/substanceinfo/100.004.986.

4. "BHA," EWG's Skin Deep, www.ewg.org/skindeep/ingredients/700740-BHA; "Butylated Compounds," Campaign for Safe Cosmetics, www.safecosmetics.org/chemicals/butylated-compounds.

5. Tasha Stoiber, "What Are Parabens, and Why Don't They Belong in Cosmetics?," Environmental Working Group, April 9, 2019, www.ewg.org/what-are-parabens.

6. "Formaldehyde," EWG's Skin Deep, www.ewg.org/skindeep/ingredients/702500-FORMALDEHYDE.

7. "Iodopropynyl Butylcarbamate," EWG's Skin Deep, www.ewg.org/skindeep/ingredients/703111-IODOPROPYNYL_BUTYLCARBAMATE.

8. Peter C. Schalock et al., "American Contact Dermatitis Society Core Allergen Series: 2020 Update," *Dermatitis: Contact, Atopic, Occupational, Drug* 31, no. 5 (2020): 279–82, www.contactderm.org/UserFiles/file/American_Contact_Dermatitis_Society_Core_Allergen.2-1_v1.pdf; Irina Webb, "Phenoxyethanol in Skin Care: Consider This!," I Read Labels for You, August 15, 2023, ireadlabelsforyou.com/phenoxyethanol-beauty-products.

9. Yufei Wang and Haifeng Qian, "Phthalates and Their Impacts on Human Health," *Healthcare* 9, no. 5 (May 2021): 63, www

.mdpi.com/2227-9032/9/5/603; "Phthalates," Campaign for Safe Cosmetics, www.safecosmetics.org/chemicals/phthalates.

10. "Petrolatum, Petroleum Jelly," Campaign for Safe Cosmetics, www.safecosmetics.org/chemicals/petrolatum; "Petroleum," EWG's Skin Deep, www.ewg.org/skindeep/ingredients /755299-petroleum.

11. "Ptfe (Teflon)," EWG's Skin Deep, www.ewg.org/skindeep /ingredients/723141-PTFE_TEFLON.

12. "Talc," EWG's Skin Deep, www.ewg.org/skindeep/ingredients /706427-TALC; "Talc," Campaign for Safe Cosmetics, www .safecosmetics.org/chemicals/talc.

13. "Retinol and Retinol Compounds," Campaign for Safe Cosmetics, www.safecosmetics.org/chemicals/retinol-and -retinol-compounds.

14. Lucija Tomljenovic, "Aluminum and Alzheimer's Disease: After a Century of Controversy, Is There a Plausible Link?," *Journal of Alzheimer's Disease* 23, no. 4 (2011): 567–98, https:// journals.sagepub.com/doi/abs/10.3233/JAD-2010-101494; Daniel Krewski et al., "Human Health Risk Assessment for Aluminium, Aluminium Oxide, and Aluminium Hydroxide," *Journal of Toxicology and Environmental Health, Part B, Critical Reviews* 10, no. 1 (2007): 1–269, www.tandfonline.com/doi /abs/10.1080/10937400701597766; "Find Ingredient Reviews and Documents," Cosmetic Ingredient Review, www.cir-safety .org/ingredients; "ToxFAQs for Aluminum," Agency for Toxic Substances and Disease Registry, March 12, 2015, wwwn.cdc .gov/TSP/ToxFAQs/ToxFAQsDetails.aspx?faqid=190&toxid =34; Keele University, "Aluminum Found In Sunscreen: Could It Cause Skin Cancer?," ScienceDaily, August 13, 2007, www.sciencedaily.com/releases/2007/08/070812084458 .htm; Alain Pineau et al., "If Exposure to Aluminium in Antiperspirants Presents Health Risks, Its Content Should Be Reduced," *Journal of Trace Elements in Medicine and*

Biology 28, no. 2 (2014): 147–50, www.sciencedirect.com
/science/article/abs/pii/S0946672X13002034?via%3Dihub.

15. Vanessa Ngan, "Allergy to Benzophenone," DermNet, 2012,
https://dermnetnz.org/topics/allergy-to-benzophenone;
"Endocrine Disruptor Assessment List," European Chemicals
Agency, https://echa.europa.eu/ed-assessment; "Substance
Infocard: Octocrylene," European Chemicals Agency, https://
echa.europa.eu/substance-information/-/substanceinfo/100
.025.683; "Substance Infocard: Homosalate," European
Chemicals Agency, https://echa.europa.eu/substance
-information/-/substanceinfo/100.003.874; Changwon Yang
et al., "Avobenzone Suppresses Proliferative Activity of
Human Trophoblast Cells and Induces Apoptosis Mediated
by Mitochondrial Disruption," *Reproductive Toxicology* 81
(2018): 50–57, https://pubmed.ncbi.nlm.nih.gov/29981360.

16. "Lead and Other Heavy Metals," Campaign for Safe
Cosmetics, www.safecosmetics.org/chemicals/lead-and-other
-heavy-metals.

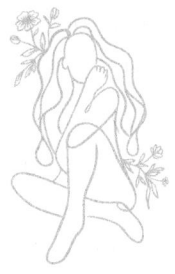

ABOUT THE AUTHOR

JORDAN LEE DOOLEY is a national bestselling author, podcast host, wife, and mama after a long struggle with recurrent pregnancy loss. Her fertility journey catapulted her into a wellness journey, where she spent years seeking answers, researching, talking to experts, and learning about ways to support her body. As she uncovered various eye-opening discoveries, she began to share her findings and experiences with her online community of hundreds of thousands of women around the world. What began as a personal quest for well-being evolved into a community-centered movement of women on a mission to do better for their bodies and families while giving God the glory.

On her podcast, *SHE,* Jordan covers wellness and womanhood from a faith-based perspective. She serves as a friend who shares what she's currently finding interesting, connects people with experts she herself is learning from, and shares some of her favorite healthy hacks and finds along the way. Check out the library of episodes at jordanleedooley.com/shownotes.

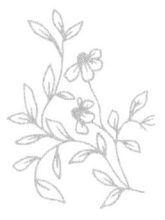

ABOUT THE TYPE

This book was set in Caslon, a typeface first designed in 1722 by William Caslon (1692–1766). Its widespread use by most English printers in the early eighteenth century soon supplanted the Dutch typefaces that had formerly prevailed. The roman is considered a "workhorse" typeface due to its pleasant, open appearance, while the italic is exceedingly decorative.

Redefine What Success Looks Like in Your Life

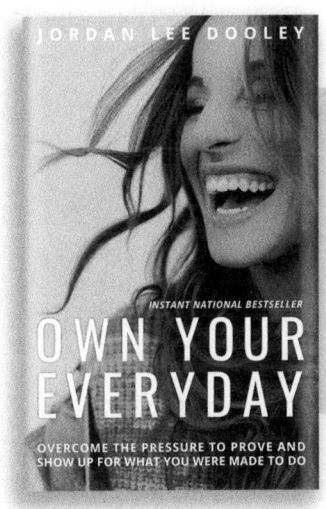

If you ever feel you need to shift your mindset but don't know how, this book will help you overcome shame, practice gratitude, and redefine success.

Learn how you can gain greater clarity about what you truly want, why you want it, and how to begin pursuing it.

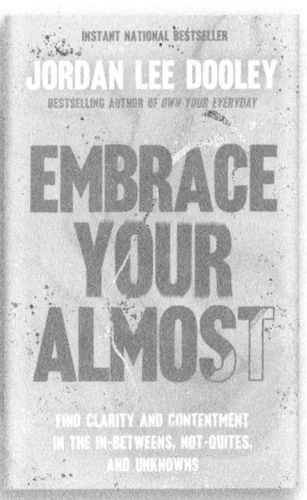

Learn more about these books at jordanleedooley.com.

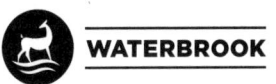